Good People Like Pot

Marijuana Revealed

MK Hall

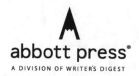

abbott press®

A DIVISION OF WRITER'S DIGEST

Abbott Press books may be ordered through booksellers or by contacting:

Abbott Press
1663 Liberty Drive
Bloomington, IN 47403
www.abbottpress.com
Phone: 1-866-697-5310

Because of the dynamic nature of the Internet, any web addresses or
links contained in this book may have changed since publication and
may no longer be valid. The views expressed in this work are solely those
of the author and do not necessarily reflect the views of the publisher,
and the publisher hereby disclaims any responsibility for them.

Any people depicted in stock imagery provided by Thinkstock are models,
and such images are being used for illustrative purposes only.
Certain stock imagery © Thinkstock.

ISBN: 978-1-4582-1575-8 (sc)
ISBN: 978-1-4582-1576-5 (e)

Printed in the United States of America.

Abbott Press rev. date: 6/9/2014

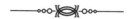

What is the worst nightmare parenting a teenager in the nineteen eighties? Losing a child to the world of illicit drugs. Pot is the enemy, the gateway drug. Nearly thirty years later it is a few years past the party bowl full of Mom and Dad's un-discarded prescription drugs. Someone's child many times over would put a handful of unknown commercial pharmaceutical drugs down their throat with a swallow of booze or Red Bull, or both.

The trends snake through all manner of manifestations. The neighbor whose Methamphetamine lab explodes, the Pot grower's house in a friend's upscale neighborhood, the busting of a drug cartel drug lord you hear about during televised news showing gunfire fighting happening in a foreign country to the south.

The Drug War is putting a dent in the everyday life of Mexicans enduring territorial drug wars, not unlike our own Alcohol Prohibition days whose Speak Easy hidden pubs, rival gang assassinations, and all out wars called "going to the mattresses" meaning shooting it out across public streets from the second story, building across from building, mattresses spread all over the floor. The gangsters put the mattresses to dual use propped in open windows as body cushion and shield when the bullets are flying, the police nowhere around. Intense deadly stuff. World wide many innocent people still die in the crossfire of such territorial drug warring.

Cartels make headlines as their leaders take control of industries and governments. Not incidentally, ten thousand Americans inside America died in 2011 as a consequence of our active Drug War. Fact stated by Jon Stewart on the Daily Show, early January, 2012.

Maybe it's time to close the gate.

During the Alcohol Prohibition many drank poison unregulated alcohol product, such as BATH TUB GIN. Bad Gin sickened and also killed people, likely as often as the mob gunfire.

Note: Red Bull is a popular energy drink popular since the late 1990s. Add 5 Hour Energy Drink, five calories? With great success they vie for the big bucks bottling two swallows of their formula in giant lipstick sized bottles sold everywhere at the checkout. For the true energy junkies legal inhalers shoot very finely powdered caffeine equal to ten cups of coffee right into an open mouth. Contra banded cocaine, even THC, the active ingredient in Cannabis, also known as Marijuana, are out in inhaler form. California.

ol4u14u14u14u14u14u14ulo

For years in the late sixties American soldiers crop dusted poison onto Marijuana crops from airplanes while flying over our South American neighbor, Columbia. Their mission was to eradicate Marihuana crops. Plant eradication has never been effective beyond the harm to the sites. It does nothing to slow the trafficking of illegal drugs. Nothing has slowed the trafficking of illegal drugs thusly lengthening the list of dire consequences. The negative results of our United States of America taxpayer supported contraband market makes a very long list.

The Federal government sprayed the poison paraquat from planes flying over growing Cannabis plants cultivated for sale, sprayed growing in Mexico. This contributed mightily to the unprecedented and hugely successful explosion of growers in America producing the American grown high grade resiny Cannabis we know today. "A little dab 'ul do ya!" Brill Cream?

Paraquat, Chemical Compound. Trade name for a long chemical name, once one of the most widely used poisons as a quick-acting killer of green plant tissue on contact. - Wikipedia November 2013. Paraquat is too dangerous for humon contact as well.

The act of willfully spending taxpayer dollars to go abroad to poison vegetation grown for American taxpayers to consume, shows a governmental scale sadistic disregard for humon well being in general and the young adults of the excessive monster Baby Boomer generation in particular.

Aside: The Baby Boomers are followed by the Millennials, the babies born from 1982 on to 2012? Millennials are another giant population mass said to be even bigger than the Baby Boomers. That ought to remove the fear of a dwindling population paying into the government as the Boomers become seniors.

Government has carte blanche to dump on Baby Boomers from the powers that be. Witness the Vietnam War. Sixty five thousand dead American servicemun. So many more damaged. You may answer for yourself if persecution by war is both then and now.

)))))))))))))))!(((((((((((((

On October 26, 2011, the Feds served notice to land owners in California to evict the lease holders off their land within forty five days if their lease holders are growing Marihuana. If there is Marihuana production in place on the land they own in forty five days the Federal Government intends to confiscate the land. Period.

The land owners had considered the state wide legality of prescription Marihuana as making their land leasers legitimate. Why did this happen? Maybe to satisfy the many other competitors for the Pot customer's dollars. The competition chooses offense as the best defense against losing greater market share to an already popular Creation Given Natural Resource Health Restorative and Superior Libation, for which no patent is possible, so far.

Cannabis, Hemp Weed, is friendly and supportive to us and our environment. It grows fast, twelve feet of root down in a year. It's deep roots protect against soil erosion. This tall potentially twelve foot tall plant is an excellent choice as an industrial fiber for many products, even as a substitute for petroleum. All besides benefits to humons consuming Cannabis.

The Supreme Court ruled mid June 2013 against patents for humon genes in a commercial testing platform because humon genes are natural basic components. One imagines a plant would be held as original material, however modified for maximum attributes. The growing processes or formulas for those maximum attributes are patentable perhaps.

Cannabis is an easily home grown flowering Herb plant that remedies a list of minor and major ailments and it's fundamentally free? A non toxic libation that isn't addictive but a preference and has no hangover? What might be the foreseeable repercussions of Marihuana's freedom? Could the lab drug pharmaceuticals, tobacco and alcohol products, illness itself, recede in popularity big time?

We live in the age of the Almighty Shareholder, a consortium of individuals, pension funds et al. Hasn't the Supreme Court endorsed corporations as people? Late 2011, about a year from our country's 2012 National Elections, corporations got the news about their person status from the Supreme Court.

January 2012, The Feds close all Cannabis dispensaries within one thousand feet of any school with a sixty day notice to move out. Denver, Colorado.

∧*∧*∧*∧*∧

"Just give it time," is the message.
"Once this work is their only choice left, we'll have plenty of American harvesters." -Karl Rowe. 2011

Those with these convictions never intend to turn their hand or bend their back to labor in a field, orchard or grove for their pay.

"God help us!" is the cry going up from farmers in Alabama and Georgia as they watch crops ruin left un-harvested. Unaccustomed Americans routinely quit field work within a day or two. Alabamians have recently set themselves apart by making it a crime to be an illegal alien in Alabama, or to employ or house one. The mass exit of undocumented foreigners is on, 2011.

This told to reveal the multi tiered demonization of both Cannabis, also known as Marihuana, and border crossing Mexicans, to increase the will of Americans to wall off our border. More exclusion. At face value, why not? Control is important.

During the Great Depression in this country, the 1930's, Mexicans were rounded up whether having American citizenship from birth or not. Trains in the state Missouri were stuffed with them to be taken to Mexico. The reason for the undocumented deportation was the idea starving whites could get the work Mexicans would have had, when there was no work.

The Marihuana Tax Act of 1937 represents the legal demonization of the Spanish word Marihuana used instead of the English word for Pot, Cannabis. Noticeably spelled Marihuana with an English sound h, not the Spanish j as in Marijuana, an authentic spelling, j pronounced h like.

Every minority in the nineteen thirties lived under the thumb of the white man's world at this time. This event of legislation codified the United States government owning major discrimination and disregard of Civil Rights.

Super news, November 7, 2012 Colorado and Washington State passed their No Penalty one ounce per adult, recreational use Pot. Recreational as in Superior Libation.

Once a person begins to look at Cannabis from an open or favorable point of view, the following question needs answering:

As legislators, if you do not support the legal use of Marihuana by responsible adults, what reason do you give for continuing criminalizing possession of Cannabis?

There is an ugly truth about Marihuana, the systematic oppression and persecution. The ultimate power of prosecution and incarceration practiced every day against individuals cultivating, buying, selling, trafficking, or possessing, Marihuana. As consumed, psycho active Hemp is not legally a crime. Contra banning Pot is based on two false premises.

First False Premise:

An individual High on Pot [in the vernacular] is turned into a criminal. How so? No deplorable or shocking behavior ensues. Society is not served removing a Cannabis ingesting individual. Not from employment, not from home, not from the public domain or local bar. There is no transgression, no call for incarceration, no decency to any punishment. Nor is any standardized distinction to be made between who is "High" and who is not to observers. Not even close. The individual benefiting from THC consumption as remedy or libation is victimized with no legitimacy. Merely naming a crime, such as contrabaning Cannabis and not looking back for substantiation when there is none, is what is criminal, a deplorable crime.

Second, Inferred, False Premise:

Cannabis is harmful. No it is not. The evidence was clear in the 1970s. Cannabis does not intoxicate, depress or by progressing degrees deteriorate an individual to unconscious or sickened on the spot, carrying a risk of making themselves a lifetime degenerate. The average beer drinking individual is running the risk of hosting a dangerous addiction to a poison. A poison that kills off vital organs, the liver and the brain, not to mention drunkards tabulate deplorable and shocking behaviors that all too frequently maim, damage or kill the innocent including babies poisoned in the womb. Many children lose their mother or father, or both, killed by a drunk person behind the wheel of a car.

Contrary to the False premises, as it happens THC, again, the active ingredient in Pot, is a key in a lock, the lock being a receptor built into all our brains. Specific THC receptors are located in the humon brain. One is located 'mainly in the central nervous system' and another receptor is 'mainly expressed in cells in the immune system'.-Wikipedia

We are born with these receptors for THC and THC only. Only Pot provides an external source for our body's THC. Study reveals long distance runners produce THC internally for their THC, tetrahydrocannabinol, receptors. This is perceived as a reward mechanism by the scientist reporting, summer 2012. It's postulated that early humons survived based on skill at running down game for food making THC a survival asset, a reward for endurance and speed.

It appears our bodies naturally produce THC in conditions long distant runners experience. Our bodies and brains treasure THC. Think Tender Healing Care. This is science.

Keep in mind Cannabis has been useful to humons as shown by written history for over five thousand years. It is part of the creation package as a Natural Resource Health Restorative, as proven by untold millions upon millions of Americans who right now are state legal twenty times over. Made legal by their state's citizens or their legislaturers voting to allow Cannabis to be prescribed by a legitimate doctor and purchased state legally. Federal law supersedes and is contrary. By adding a late 2013 codicil the Feds are likely backing off to accommodate the state legal laws reference Marihuana. Plus Washington and Colorado have legalized Pot for recreational use. The Feds need to help work out the taxation. Indications are of upcoming terms for Colorado to proceed with legal Cannabis sales with a tax.

January first 2014 saw the first day of taxed and legal Marijuana sales to all comers in Colorado. The lines were long in Denver and the price escalated through the day due to supply and demand principles. The tourists were dismayed to discover themselves frozen out of a legal place to light up. Until the café's are in place as smoking bars in a few months they are out of luck. The hotels say no marihuana use allowed, and it has to be private land to inhale. Imagine ads in the paper renting out your parlor at say, thirty dollars an hour? Could that be?

As summer 2013 ends we grow hopeful with another state going medical Marihuana legal. There are drips and drabs of a looming tipping point to legalization on a Federal scale. A Texas border county Sheriff bemoans his budget squeeze. Says he must spend in his county and forego catching every bag of Cannabis carrying individual coming across the border into his county.

Hot and wet is our summer, 2013. Weather-wise. Maybe the Gay rights movement's recent burst forward to greater equality is giving momentum to basic truth and justice. Liberty, Justice, and Equality Together Make Freedom.

∧∧∧∧∧∧∧∧∧∧∧∧∧∧∧∧∧∧∧∧∧∧∧∧∧∧∧∧∧

Attorney General Eric Holder alluded to an upcoming statement of new policy reference the taxing issue in Colorado for legal Cannabis sales. New Policy Statement forthcoming in a few months. This stated in early June, 2013, United States Senate, during a routine hearing.

Talk of prison sentences being disproportionately long is afoot, early August, 2013.

The terms have been spoken by Eric Holder. The initial description includes asking the Federal Prosecutors in the legalizing states and DC to respect the state's law and not prosecute the newly freed to buy Pot, Pot liking people. The District of Columbia voted Yes to the medical Marihuana issue three years ago and are only now getting the mechanism to implement. Congress decides these things for the people of the District of Columbia in practice, it seems.

By March the ridiculously all cash Pot sale business legally conducted in Colorado has more than tripled the income expectations for the state coffers. All Cash. Colorado's bankers remain frigid, holding out for Federal Legality. Imagine the ponderous problem of unbankable cash. That would seem to open the door for another kind of business known as money laundering. Why not design a new bank taking cash. A consortium from the Pot industry itself could do it.

Legal Pot would have to mean truly legal Pot so there can be investor confidence in the new world of Cannabis production and merchandizing. A Cannabis industry is gearing up big time. Cigarette manufacturers are getting in the picture with product planning. Legitimate gadgets are set for expanding sales. All see massive profits in their future. Food with exact THC potencies await us.

YES WE CANNABIS! That is the title given the Cover story published in the April 8, 2013 issue on Page 67 of Fortune Magazine. Entrepreneurs are seeking investors as investors seek Cannabis ventures all about and around Cannabis production and consumption and gear.

These states; [see the list of twenty states, pages 111 to 113 this book]. These states give their Citizens the right to purchase and consume Marihuana medicinally due to the people of each of those states getting their amendment or referendum on the ballot and getting it passed or having state legislators informed enough to pass legalization for medicinal use. It's medical Marijuana for eighteen of the twenty, with two states, Washington and Colorado, approving Recreational use, too. Not anywhere else in America so far.

The District of Columbia has also approved Medical Marihuana. People in Florida are offering a petition to put medical Marihuana to a vote November, 2014. The Referendum has been targeted for a court case. State Attorney General Pam Bondi saying the referendum will be misleading to the public on the ballot. News early November, 2013. The trend to tolerance should trump her initiative. January 2014 the petitions to legalize are numerous and the original one, People for Medical Marijuana, already has many more than required in February.

February 2014 the court ruled to allow the vote for Medical Marihuana to be on the Florida 2014 ballot.

duhduhduhduhduhduhduhduhduhduh

There is no lethal dose of Marihuana. Caffeine as in coffee, cola, and chocolate, some pain killer pills, causes receptors to grow in our brains so our brains will receive caffeine. Caffeine is legal, addictive, and lethal in a large enough dose, per all scientific harm indexing. Marijuana typically consumed is trustworthily harmless. No evidence exists to prove otherwise in any general, persuasive or noticeable way.

Let's take the good stuff away from the sellers of other contraband. Allow adults to buy Marihuana legally. It's only fair. Close the gate to the hard drugs a pusher would push. Why not find Marihuana contrabanding law invalid and unenforceable, severing it from the law as is offered to do in the law itself. See the legal options to legalize contained here in this book, beginning page 212.

Consider, when a law is deemed legally unconstitutional that means it was always legally unconstitutional. Restitution could be in order.

Recommended good start: Our President pardons all offenders charged with only Marihuana offense(s). That should have the immediate effect of keeping all former offenses surrounding Marijuana to effectively be off the books, no longer in effect. Persecution ends.

No more Pot arrests. Huge public opinion supporting this change required. It could spread to cause the undoing of the requirement within treaties the USA has with many nations to prosecute, having persecuted, their populaces over Marihuana.

November 5, 2013 Attorney General Eric Holder announces his opinion the sentencing guidelines in place offer exaggerated sentencing. He wants new transition to life outside programs to go in place and release of those who qualify. Prison over crowding is so great that if all the mandatory sentences being served were cut in half the over crowding would still be twenty five percent too much. An ongoing story no doubt.

May 18, 2013, a consortium of South American diplomats conclude their countries may well be better served legalizing Cannabis. They cite Uruguay studying to do just that at present. The newest President of Mexico is calling for legalization, June 2013.

December 2013 Uruguay legalized for residents only.

Imagine the healing that will take place once we earn respect world wide by finally claiming our divisive and deviant legislative acts for what they are. We must cease pushing the criminal creation of lawlessness around the globe. Pot decriminalization will likely transform our country as the truth does and give us back our place as leaders of the free world by right of deed as in a good deed.

One in five of us use tobacco. One third or more of all tobacco users will die of tobacco use. That makes tobacco account for about one tenth of all deaths, everyday, every year, every hour. That many deaths have tobacco use as cause on their death certificate or should. Multiply that number to show those harmed by second hand tobacco and this drug is both menace and mass killer. Whereas Marihuana is an easily grown non addictive Creation Given Natural Resource, Health Restorative and Superior Libation. Besides being an asset to the humon condition physically, mentally and emotionally, Cannabis as Hemp has many uses as an asset to industry and the envirnment.

There is no fatal amount to imbibe of Cannabis.
Science has proven you cannot die from a Marijuana overdose. NO death by Cannabis. No toxins are present in this Herb. Witness the non criminal Cannabis partakers near and far. Have you heard how Cannabis is valuable to those in cancer treatment? See normal people. Nor is it possible to distinguish which is which, who is who among us, Pot user or non Pot user? Our culture uses urine tests and sniffer dogs to make the distinction. Our culture also provides a formula for defeating the urine tests as well. One

purchases a drink that "cleanses" the pot from one's urine with some abstinence plus drinking this drink. Golden Seal is good for same used routinely, to some degree. Which impugns the entire false assumption that applicants pass a urine test for the employer to satisfy the employer's liability insurer. Liability details per Cannabis are given nowhere.

Testing urine as a gateway to equal opportunity employment is a farce, a criminal farce, an Equal and Civil Rights offence.

Watch for a Pharmaceutical Empire funded study of a small group, less than forty individuals, divided as heavy vs. non Pot people for a broad conclusion of late life loss of 'motivation'(?) assigned to the Pot people. Hmmm. Hardly criminal, if verifiable. The concluded 'loss of motivation' as terminology is based on the said to be observed lower dopamine levels in the brains of the Pot heads. Perhaps a second control group of lifetime meditators would match the Pot people? Thus perhaps indicating whose chemicals really win?

%#%#%#%

Real Life Case in Point:

A man loses his job to lay off in November 2009. In January, 2010 he gets hired to work in his chosen field at a lesser job. He is on the job working on Monday after his pee test on Friday. He is let go that first day for having flunked his pee test, even with weeks of abstinence, tripped up perhaps by inadvertent unanticipated dehydration which concentrates any THC.

He continues on unemployment. One year later, February 2011, he is hired at his career former level of expertise, only now at half pay due to the economic downturn hitting the construction industry so hard. This employer, no drug test. He would remain at his job if the pressures of his bosses, a married couple, if their personal lives and the economic stresses in the construction industry had not precipitated his lay off October 11, 2012, one year and eight months after being hired. Update: He's back working with the now single former employer, the husband.

Who is there to defend the everyday persecution by arrest for Marihuana possession? Not the knowledgeable. But indeed, lots of Big Business Industries are riding the criminalization of this practical vegetation. Marijuana can't be patented. We the public are to legally make do with the lab versions of THC delivery to those receptors for THC in our brains.

The synthetics, no thank you. The synthetics have failed the public miserably and made our United States Congress chase whatever new formula's latest offensive ingredient is to make it illegal.

The overhead and harm of the "War on Drugs" is unending and unfathomable. Unending, so far. The facts will soon speak for themselves drowning out the lies once and for all.

Share this book. Speak up. Vote knowledgeably.

Imagine: Could it be that our body's self healing mechanisms turn on with THC? Let's find out for a fact! If only Americans could be permitted to do an up to date scientific study of THC.

As it turns out, the reason we have no studies to find out the positives and negatives of Pot as consumed by people is simple. The Federal Food and Drug Administration is very stingy with the permits to do so. It requires that any participants be experienced users of Pot and that they submit to living in a hospital for the duration of the permitted study. This revealed by a top oncologist in California on National Public Radio speaking with a Food and Drug Administration, the FDA, representative for a back and forth discussion of the merits or menace of Pot. The practicing medical doctor wants his cancer patients to be part of the non criminalized population. He offered consistently convincing anecdotal, factual and statistical evidence in favor of allowing the studying of Marihuana to proceed vigorously and did prevail over the more irrelevant assertions made to keep Pot demonized. The oncologist doctor, the NPR radio broadcast interviewee mentioned here, has great credentials as the head oncologist in his southern California hospital. He admitted he himself has enjoyed the benefits of Pot all through his own adult life.

Pregnant? Marihuana does not pass into the baby through the placenta. Baby is not getting any effect from THC. Mothers are relieved of the hard pains of the birth and may have nice pregnancies aided by Cannabis, rich in Herbal ingredients. So many humon conditions make use of THC as asset. We deserve as inquiring informed people to find out all Pot's attributes as they benefit the humon condition. We are not meant to go on ignorantly ignoring the importance and value of what we call psycho active Hemp.

CCDDCCDDCCDDCCDDCCDDC

This is a country of people routinely pledging allegiance to Liberty and Justice for all. It is an offense to all thinkers, scientists and people of logic everywhere to persist in arcane ignorance.

Keeping a population held back by bad law will ultimately back fire. Besides, who isn't ready to see our people learning how to care for themselves, staving off illnesses while maybe cutting health care costs individual by individual. Perhaps allowing the health care industry to grow more able in sophisticated ways to care for the sick. The alternative might be the breaking down of our health care system under overwhelming stretching thin of ever more unaffordable health care provider services. Suppose Pot is the ingredient needed to transform the basic platform of humon health?

Learn this fact: The Herb Cannabis has been shown in written and oral history over the last thousands of years of civilization to be an asset to the humon condition. It's time to right the wrong of criminalization.

~~~~~~~~~~~~~~~~~~~~~

The Humon Story as it unfolds:

Folks in Key West in the first decade of the last century bought their Cannabis scooped from a bin, wrapped in paper and sold by weight. It sold in pharmacies. Doctors recommended it.

In Jamaica families with Cannabis and children were found to thrive. This from a published study in the 1980's as reported by NORML [National Organization for the Reform of Marihuana Law].

The family's thriving remains true if a family remains beyond the Jamaican national government's reach of implementation of a commitment to our United States government to criminalize Cannabis as contraband. The report seemed also to say when Ganja dealing is a part of the parent's lives, the family thrives as well. During the time of the study Cannabis was commonly used to dissipate suffering from asthma. The youngsters who were found to partake of Cannabis in their early adolescence grew up as well adjusted as comparable Cannabis free children in the over ten years of the study.

In the nineteen seventies the many historical facts and truths surrounding Hemp were given to the good people of this country by way of the formally hugely popular and commonly known still renown organization, NORML, The National Organization for the Reform of Marihuana Law. Other sources were publications. High Times Magazine, an ongoing enterprise, with it's wonderful pictures of resin drenched psycho active Hemp. Still going is Common Cause, look on-line. Plus at least one TV special aired on the Public Broadcasting System in the early nineteen nineties in the greater Miami area on WLRN TV. It may have been hosted by a young Asian American. His hour long special programming addressed the history of Marihuana. See also The Nature of Desire, another old Public Broadcasting System special re-aired. Cannabis is one of the three plant subjects. Very informative. More later.

~~~~~~~~~~~~~~~~~~~~~~~

The legally created by constitutional amendment prohibition against alcohol was repealed with another United States Constitution Amendment after thirteen years. The stated motivation for the Alcohol Prohibition was Cirrhosis. Cirrhosis of the liver is almost epidemic. Much more moving was the resonating need to end drunken husbands and fathers harming their families.

The catalyst for repealing? Mothers from Michigan's waterfront. Their waterfront became importation central for booze from Canada. Michigan Mothers marched in

Washington D.C. to the Whitehouse seeking regulation of alcohol to stop the preying of bootleggers on their elementary school age children.

Those Michigan Lake alcohol importers were the first big winner contraband drug pushers. The Michigan mothers claimed their children were getting drunk while at school.

Alcohol bootleggers were joyfully selling booze as a contraband drug to the American masses for thirteen years ending in 1933. Alcohol drug dealers made so very much extraordinary wealth selling contraband booze they sought to have a Congress to provide another legislated contraband drug market and spent enough money to make it so. We got the Narcotics Tax Act of 1937.

Our Congresses in the 1930s were notorious and publicly known for corruption. Some legislators were prosecuted for their individual corruption while a legislator.

Implementation of Punishment reference the Narcotics or Marihuana Tax Act of 1937 meant arresting those who had failed to pay the tax on the Pot they are handling. Proof of having paid the tax had to be on hand if law enforcement caught you. Yet no one was licensed to collect the tax on commercial Pot. It became an unlicensed narcotic, contraband, for not having the right document to prove a tax is paid. Quickly Marihuana went underground. The same as the original Harrison Tax Act of 1914 criminalizing opiates and morphine, only now Marihuana is added to list. This time minorities became exclusively targeted.

Score a victory for the Bad Guys. They successfully created and implemented an unregulated mucho nefarious underworld. Being the professionals they are, thugs targeted neighborhood after neighborhood. Pushers amplified the scale of criminal activity obtaining results that can only exist when a law excludes and bans for legal sale what is addictive and harmful. Pot is neither. Dangerous drugs foisted on an unsuspecting public with no regulation or consumer protections birthed illegal drug cartels and whole communities are brought to their knees. One example is Liberty City in Miami, Florida. Mid nineteen eighties even the police wouldn't go there routinely.

The money stream to the Bad Guys pockets' is wide and deep and gets wider still to this day. We the public are caught in the middle as the Bad Guys stealthily grow their business. Often that middle is a no man's land fraught with live gunfire in a thug territorial battle.

Pain killer prescription drugs selling illegally rule.

Cocaine and Heroin, are a dealer's dream, great for client retention. They may well stay addicted until they hit bottom and start over or die. Each of Cocaine and Heroin is staging a comeback or conquering a new country even now, late 2013.

Early 2014 the focus on keeping Americans unable to acquire massive quantities of commercial pharmaceutical laboratory painkiller pills sold illegally has resulted in a huge up tick in opiate addicted customers. Squeeze the Balloon.

Pushers Push. Vendors vend. Government could serve us better giving opiates away with direct compassionate contact, non judgmental interaction, factual. In a generation illicit nasty drugs could be history, virtually gone.

The present is grueling for those on the frontlines of this Drug War. In the end, a tiny percentage of us choosing the 'drug' route would function with everyone else. Such product made available in routine commerce. No inappropriate marketing. Sales never judgmental. Interactions based on compassion.

Some War, the Drug War.

cvbcvbcvbcvbcvbcvbc

The Harrison Tax Act of 1914 got the ball rolling for codifying 'drugs' as contraband by the United States Congress. The Act passed against vociferous protesting from the American Medical Association. Congress decided against allowing doctors to maintain and treat hard drug addicts. It had taken from 1908 to 1914 to get the Harrison Act passed making the sale of morphine and heroin, opiates, illegal.

Immediately use tripled. In a few months the problem had morphed. This because the underworld is far better at widely proliferating and distributing illegal drugs than regulated caring doctors prescribing them.

It's one hundred years later, 2014. Enough is enough. It took one hundred and thirty six years to get the endorsement of slavery off the books. Let's stop the misapplication of tax payer funds doing no more than persecuting innocent people, the consumer. Enforce freedom instead. Help and understanding are better solutions than punishment.

- **per·se·cute** [púrssə kyŞt](*past and past participle* **per·se·cut·ed**, *present participle* **per·se·cut·ing**, *3rd person present singular* **per·se·cutes**) *vt*
- **oppress people:** to systematically subject a race or group of people to cruel or unfair treatment, e.g. because of their ethnic origin or religious beliefs
- **pester somebody:** to make somebody the victim of continual pestering or harassment

Encarta ® World English Dictionary © & (P) 1998-2005 Microsoft Corporation. All rights reserved.

The American Medical Association, caught off guard by the last minute inclusion of Marihuana as a narcotic in the

Narcotics Tax Act of 1937, still managed to mount a presence of descent before it passed.

After the Harrison Act of 1914 and the Narcotics Tax Act of 1937 comes our current multi illicit drug related United States Congressional Acts, numbering in the thirties, each an add on done chronologically beginning after the update done in 1970; Title: Drug Abuse and Control-1970 Law.

Following is a chronological list of all the Acts of Congress included in this Title or Congressional Act, all put into action tax payer funded. By action read studies, reports, meetings and field work as set up by and reporting to and over seen by an assigned congressional committee.

Those brought in to do the work are whole auspices like the Coast Guard or FDA etc. The list of Acts reads like a march through time. A news making headline referencing an illicit or about to be illicit drug becomes a legislator's answer back with fresh, inconsequential in the larger scheme of things as any sort of prevention, one Congressional Act after another. Severely consequential when a felony conviction hits an individual and family, and causes prison crowding and the near impossible challenges to former inmates in the aftermath of prison life.

Currently Marihuana has the distinction of a Schedule I Drug Classification in the United States of America. It defies the imagination how these requirements for a 'drug' to be Schedule I, 1) the worst for abuse, 2) lacking medical applications and 3)showing no level of safe consumption, do not exempt Pot.

Keep in mind the 'Pot is Good Theory' initially caught the minds and imaginations of mainstream people when the news media covered the story of cancer victims getting their appetites back formerly lost to debilitating nausea caused by Chemotherapy. Yes! Medicinal Pot Efficacy!

No possible match to allow for inclusion of Marihuana in the three required characteristics to be a Schedule I Felonious Drug Classification. The project to keep Americans intimidated and cowed is a success. We are about eighty years along in an unrelenting march of lies brought to us by the media and put into existence by our government in the hands of big business working both the government and the media.

Remember the Doctor selected for Surgeon General whose big flaw foiling his acceptance at the time was saying he believes Marihuana has medicinal attributes? Dr. Bork, was it? Renown for brilliance, turned down by speaking truth.

Early eighties. It appears this take on history has been rewritten.

Only one organized group, The American Medical Association, the AMA, protested to Congress the inclusion of Marihuana in the 1937 Tax Act. Now not so much. They are pill prescribers nowadays, possessing little to no knowledge of any natural remedies including nutrition. This is changing. It appears monkind is more interested in taking charge of it's own individual bodies with responsible choices of late.

Public relations in order to swing the buying public one way or another often gives the truth short shift. The 1930's movie Reefer Madness shows couples gathering in a living room to party. After a bit of Reefer, things fall apart and one individual appears bent on homicidal mania.

He's shown running madly down the middle of the street.

The ensuing mayhem as portrayed in the movie bases itself on a major tragedy of the day unrelated to Marihuana, but used as such to persuade aversion to Pot in front of Congress. See the Anslinger story in later pages.

Pfizer Pharmaceuticals produced the movie "Reefer Madness" for general release in theaters. It's out on VHS tape, maybe DVD. In the early nineteen thirties Pfizer had a patent on Bayer Aspirin. Dumping on the competition in the movie theater helped ensure the success of Pfizer's over the counter pain killer newly launched, Bayer Aspirin.

Marihuana was seen as competition, being simply Created. Not Patentable. Cannabis and Hemp are thrown aside. Enter Big Oil.

Never mind the huge Pharmaceutical Empire made a second third and forth foray into producing a lab Cannabis, imitation Marihuana, that looks like vegetation. They also produced, deemed ineffective, THC pills.

The name for the original imitation vegetation Pot is K2. It's not a pill, it closely resembles the real Pot vegetation. It's sold over the counter. Front page, December 12, 2011, in the Monday Tampa Tribune, is an update relating to K2, billed as a Novelty Drug. Apparently due to adverse effects some of it's previous ingredients caused, those ingredients have been legislated as contraband. K2's current newest ingredient list product is out and getting even worse reviews for causing even more threatening psychotic episodes. There are reports of folks firing their gun at "monsters". It's sending people to the hospital in greater numbers than the original K2.

October 2012, the sale of synthetic Pot may be over. It certainly proved harmful. It's hard to improve on some things. For instance the easily grown weed, Ganja. It's a Natural Resource Health Restorative also known as Cannabis or Pot. By any name, an asset to humons. No overdose deaths possible.

Lately Ketamine, the horse tranquillizer, that's also humon contraband, has come into favor as a balancer for some actual humon beings' disorders. Some adolescents are able to live normally taking it. More normal than ever before.

Back to the article on K2, the original synthetic Pot.

It also told of a bath salts drug mostly available for purchase on line. Bath Salts? The manufacturers of drugs are all out ready and able to produce and sell their new patented Legal Drug alternatives to satisfy demand for drugs. Legislators do a merry chase playing catch up as the casualty statistics mount up on Big Pharmaceutical's and little independent producer's efforts to capture some of the Cannabis market with a patented lab drug.

What is the FDA doing anyway? Perhaps in late summer 2012 Congress changed the rules, no more synthetic Pot.

THC is the active ingredient of the four hundred twelve or so chemical components making Marihuana, Marihuana. Not a single one of the four hundred some odd components are toxic. All humons, all humon brains are made complete with built in receptors for THC, TetraHydroCanabinol, exclusively THC receptors, and Cannabis is the obvious choice. By the way, humon brains grow receptors for caffeine. Caffeine does have a lethal harm index.

Obviously, before the nineteen seventies The Narcotics Tax Act of 1937 passed Congress and made Marihuana contraband. The 1937 law was implemented against i.e. arresting only, Black, Hispanic or Latino and Latinas, and Asian people. Marijuana arrests became the means of systematic persecution by prosecution and the threat of prosecution for minorities.

A spring 2013 aired remark by an incumbent legislator: "At the time the law {Narcotics Tax Act of 1937} passed, nobody {in this country} was smoking Pot, anyway."

It appears he meant the governing public of the day, the insulated and isolated White Anglo Saxon Protestants. They were isolated from Pot.

Arresting people for Marihuana possession after it's inclusion in the 1937 Narcotics Tax Act became a great tool of oppression. The Act's enforcement waited to become an equal opportunity tool of oppression beginning at the kick off of the "Just Say No" Campaign. Thank you, Mrs. Ronald Regan, 1987.

At the time, a Miami policeman said this on camera about cocaine users, "We may not be able to catch them when they steal, but we can catch them with their 'drugs'." Thereby oversimplifying while endorsing the commonly held notion of the day that a 'Drug' addiction makes thieves of it's users in order to satisfy their expensive 'drug' addiction, no exceptions. The demonizing of 'Drugs' and it's users reached it's first peaking and so did use.

Running the price up on the street value of cocaine is seen as positive from an enforcement point of view. No doubt the criminals selling it agree. The cocaine thugs responded to the free publicity from the "Just Say No" Campaign by turning cocaine into cheaper Crack cocaine, thereby greatly enlarging their client base. The thugs upped the number of Americans addicted to cocaine a quantum leap with crack.

The "JUST SAY NO" campaign was designed for elementary aged children in Miami in the late eighties. Believe it. This brings to mind a youngster in fourth grade turning down his young counterpart fringe element fellow child's offer to take a free sample taste.

This is ludicrous. We passed laws. No selling within one thousand feet of a school to that child pusher. That's an automatic jail term. Three strikes and You are Out!

Translation: Three felony convictions accumulated? Incarceration without parole forever for you. Many may have been scared straight but even more truly, would be productive individuals, are now jailed all too often in too many instances in well beyond humone prison capacity conditions, and are there for life.

Think of the derelict and vagrant Vietnam War veteran alcoholic living on the street who is picked up twice and receives a felony conviction each time for walking out of the same convenience store with a six pack of beer. That's two strikes. This is a true story. In this case the felon is back as a successful citizen of excellence for well over fifteen years. So happy ending. This veteran had near by family and friends to help pave the way back.

Children of middle and high school age were taken from their schools to see the inside of a prison as a field trip designed to scare them 'straight', as in 'Drug' free.

November, 2012 it appears releasing some victims of the three strikes sentencing law will be released due to serving excessive time incarcerated for their offenses.

Humonity awakens? Right here in the U.S. of A.?

∧∧*∧*∧*∧*

The 'Drug' problem keeps morphing it's way along to whatever tune of nasty 'Drug' song the underworld feels like serving up. Many prisons are built by taxpayers and filled to over flowing. We have the 'honor' of imprisoning two point two million Americans mid 2013. That is, we imprison more of our own by percentage than any other country, bar none, even China. And our prisoners are substantially slave labor. We allow outside contractors to have prison labor working in prison. It keeps costs down while knocking the air out of un-imprisoned labor pricing. In Louisiana a humongous prison produces commercial products on site.

They farm extensively and do lots of animal husbandry.

On another tier we taxpayers pay to attempt to keep prisoners from remaining as Kingpins of Gangs in the 'Drug' Business while in lock up, incarcerated. We keep failing.

Trained dogs can smell a cell phone even if it's in a vat of oil. That's intense effort on both side's part. Makes you wonder. This fact was found in a New Yorker Magazine article. A Sniffer Dog's ability works because cell phones have a unique odor, we are told. Inmates hide the cell phones they use to stay connected with their gang members who are on the outside. Not happening or not news worthy any more.

We are well into the twenty first century and more than seventy years into THE POT WAR. A victory means toppling the head of a marginal portion of the contraband 'Drug' industry or dismantling a sophisticated underground tunnel with large carts filled with contraband Cannabis moving on tracks from a warehouse in Mexico to a warehouse in California.

All while knowing full well the demand for the contraband is what seals the deal on continuing the sale of Cannabis. Picture all that unfathomable untaxed wealth flowing to the underworld. Marihuana is our country's biggest cash crop, bigger than corn, circa pre ethanol.

One out of fifteen American high schoolers in a study reported smoking Pot on a daily basis. This on NPR, National Public Radio, airing December 14, 2011. Early 2014 we hear about the reduction in teenage alcohol consumption.

Archeological digs have experts concluding a long ago culture had a special round room for the birthing of babies. Cannabis burned in special crevices in the wall during births. Science tells us the placenta does not allow passage of any Cannabinols to baby. Mothers to be do well with Pot as a medicinal Herb tea. Our first President, George Washington, grew quantities of Hemp at Mount Vernon. Hemp is a natural rope fiber. It was grown for Naval purposes in our mid west regions. Hemp has many applications from rope to stopping the erosion of our land.

The PSYCHO ACTIVE VARIETY OF CANNABIS, aka MARIHUANA, Weed, Hemp, Ganja, Grass, Pot, Cannabis etc.

PREVENTS GLACOMA

ACTS AS ANULGESIC, ANTIHISTIMINE & EXPECTERANT

RELAXES OR ENERGIZES

RELIEVES NAUSEA

RELIEVES ANXIETY

SHARPENS MENTAL FOCUS

IMPROVES EYESIGHT

REDUCES SUFFERING

AIDS SOCIALIZING

ENHANCES EXERCISE

ENCOURAGES CREATIVITY

INCREACES APPETITE

AUGMENTS LAUGHTER, _THE_ BEST MEDICINE!

& MARIHUANA APPEARS TO LOWER BLOOD PRESSURE AND BOOST THE IMMUNE SYSTEM

See list of specific illnesses Marijuana remedies page 196.

^^*^*^*^*^*^*^*^*^*^*^*^*

For hundreds of years ending about three hundred years ago the people of continental Europe including Italy, plus Great Britain did not eat tomatoes. Tomatoes, it was widely known, were fine as ornamentals but not for eating because everyone knew them to be poisonous. Eventually a King did eat a tomato, enjoyed it and lived.

Note: Profiles; The King's Meal, by L. Collins, published by the New Yorker Magazine Nov. 21, 2011 mentions on page sixty nine "Tomatoes---known as 'apples of love'---had been in England since the sixteenth century, but people didn't start eating them until around 1800." Perhaps it was King George III of the House of Hanover, The English King 1760-1820.

DO YOU EAT RED SPAGITTI SAUCE, SALSA, BBQ?

In 2010, one point six million people were arrested for Marihuana offenses in America. One million, 2011. For decades nearly seventy percent of all those incarcerated were serving time on a 'Drug' related Felony conviction. Maybe less of a percentage now. Now we have 'Drug' court to alleviate the overwhelmed courts. We pay for a whole auxiliary court system to streamline the ushering of the there to be convicted alleged 'Drug' felons and misdemeanor perps aka perpetrators, who are booked into the Judicial System over 'Drugs'.

It's a shame logic was not employed to understand that the overwhelming numbers clogging the system of justice meant we were arresting the innocent, those not belonging in our jails and courts. No Just Cause in place. We currently also share the shame of incarcerating those with mental illnesses and disabilities inappropriately housed in our jails in large numbers.

This was published in a subsidiary of the Tampa Tribune Newspaper MARCH 8,2011 HIGHLANDS TODAY, (Daily

Newspaper Serving Highlands County, Florida), PAGE 2, STORY TITLED <u>POLICE SERVE NARCOTICS SEARCH WARRANT</u>. The Story:

Do to an on going investigation, we are told, and a neighbor's complaint of "activity", police raid a City of Avon Park free standing house to find a trace amount of Marihuana and 'Drug' paraphernalia. Therefore the police made a misdemeanor arrest for the trace amount of Pot, and a felony charge for the possession of the 'Drug' paraphernalia. That individual is taken to jail on the spot.

Proper authorities are to be notified because toddlers are in the house along with three adults. A relative having walked over to the house, is arrested for an outstanding warrant for a failure to appear for a court date on unrelated 'Drug' charges.

Is that how we make a better neighborhood? What is the rest of the story? Are the lives of those five adults and three little children being set on a path to betterment? We may only wonder. It's worth mentioning that the stated goal of the County Sheriff of virtually crime free Highlands County is to make Highlands County in Florida 'Drug' free. 'Drug', i.e. contraband, free. Maybe that qualifies as an ongoing investigation.

Never mind. Florida was 2011's Go-To state for the grossly huge amounts of prescription drugs supplying the nation's illicit, not properly prescribed legitimately laboratory made, pain killer drugs. Lab-made prescription pain killers are the latest drug choice to abuse, 2011. It doesn't get the word drug surrounded by apostrophizes because it is in actuality legally lab produced pain killer pills like oxycodin that are being abused. Regular legal drugs from the local drug store receive no special emphasis of contraband to be voiced or written.

Prescribed pills are in demand for abuse. Not usually counterfeit pills either, the real deal from big name pharmaceuticals. Slowly the ability to trace back the supply chain emerges. The punishing of those who handed out five hundred pills at a time to an individual? Not so much. The punishing of the supplying manufactures? Didn't make the news if it happened.

The earlier referenced article in the paper about the cops entering an Avon Park, Florida home to make a very early morning bust includes a photo taken of a City of Avon Park Detective exiting the Pot arrestee's house. The Highlands Today newspaper photographer came to the arrest location as it unfolded to get the picture. The caption gave the alleged perpetrators house's street name and revealed it as in the 300 block. So much for small town news worthiness and the rights of individuals. Once the arrests are official they will be published in the paper with names, addresses and the charges. (Update; Local Journalism has dropped it's aforementioned format of arrests coverage.)

Let's recap the activity in this actual event. A person goes to jail to be booked for criminal possession of a legally purchased pipe? Rolling papers? A bong? An empty baggie with tiny bits of Pot as evidence, the trace amount? Because of the association with the alleged perpetrator's misdemeanor trace amount of Marihuana those otherwise legal items turn into contraband, felonious possession contraband. A man is arrested. Do you suppose this arrested individual will have a lawyer that subpoenas the proof of the mentioned investigation that allows for the Narcotic Search Warrant served in the early morning, house occupants caught unawares? By now we all know that possession of Marihuana, even consumption of Marihuana, poses no threat to the individual or others. Witness the nineteen, now twenty, states plus Washington DC, whose people have the advantage of legal, if the Feds don't butt in, prescription medical Marihuana.

Postscript. Perhaps unrelated to the March, 2011 arrest outlined above in Avon Park, Florida: In October 2012 a finished transition took place changing the Avon Park Police Department policemun into Highlands County Sheriff's Department Officers, without their last Police Force Captain. The picture in the paper showed a very proud group of fifteen mun.

)&*^&)(&*^&)(&*^&)(&*^&)(&*^&(

Holland? Uruguay? Portugal? Perhaps the leaders of Uruguay have implemented their novel idea for turning their 'Drug' issues around. They said they'd allow everyone to grow their own. Holland, imbibe at a Pot sold for consumption Café. Portugal, eleven years ago legalized public consumption of 'drugs' in general to calm the violence down. It worked.

Worldwide, there is not one place, except one's own domicile, or any privately owned or rented place with a tolerant persuasion, where, you are privately ensconced sufficiently, where one may smoke Pot entirely legally. Portugal kept their laws naming drugs contraband and lost the day to day implementation of the law. They simply stopped arresting the citizens of Portugal for 'drugs'.

Criminal possession, with or without the intention to sell does vary in legality place to place.

Uruguay is moving on allowing an individual six Pot plants while encouraging mini cooperatives with up to forty eight plants. And commercial growers are about to become legal, too.

Travel can be a time of abstinence for Potheads, or not.

A quality accommodation respects one's privacy if the occupant takes reasonable precautions against being obtrusive. Even to hide in a bathroom, fanny fan on, or sneak somewhere, it's a risk, September, 2013, Florida.

Movies help spread the notion of the innocence of Cannabis to the many. So who knows? Freedom <u>may</u> exist on private land and structures, owners permitting or unaware.

No actual consequences from law enforcement exist for anyone in America for having smoked. Flunking a perspective employer's pee screening test doesn't mean an arrest.

Choose a privately owned or rented space, owners permitting, for Pot consumption. A safe Pot party? In Colorado, maybe. January 16,2013.

Do to Policy, a DUI, Driving Under the Influence, arrest is a potential outcome if you are driving and something involving the police ensues. Regional and local variables apply.

@#@@#@@#@@#@@#@

Did you see HBO television's Nurse Jackie demonstrate the raw apple turned pipe with a knife and straw? She made the pipe for a character in the HBO TV show series of the same name. The character for whom the pipe is made is given it as the character's salvation from his cancer treatment's side effect of, in his case, advanced nausea. Rx Pot. Nurse Jackie in TV script shortcut style volunteers the ambulance driver character in the show is all set to be the cancer treatment out patient's dealer. That's beyond basic cable television fare.

Pipes. So normal and informed to be allowed what's graced pipes since time immemorial, since pipes.

Take a fat straw cut to about four inches, wrap in aluminum foil shaping a crater like bowl at one end extending past the straw with the foil. Perhaps leave a portion of the straw at the mouth end exposed. Fashion a screen with a small square of doubled foil large enough to form the bottom of the bowl and to also cover over the outside of the bowl somewhat. Punch a good number of pin holes in the bowl bottom. Viola`, a pipe.

Cultivation, selling and buying are each illegal everywhere on earth with a government, mid 2013. Quantities to punishments vary. Yes, the licensed places in Holland sell and people imbibe with impunity on site. Set quantities are tolerated some places. Yes, a stadium full of revelers and sports enthusiasts in Texas have turned their stadium into a haze of Pot smoke through out football games on occasion. Yes, the billion plus dollars spent on Cannabis annually makes Cannabis the biggest cash crop in the USA historically. Corn competes.

California is being selectively regulated by the Feds, October 8, 2011. They are breaking up the big Pot selling franchising storefronts saying they sell to those without a prescription too. Prescription Pot is available for purchase from the many smaller storefronts in California and they will persist.

The Cannabis War will end and the people will have won.

This could happen based on the introduction of compassion by humons for humons in general. We need each other, and ourselves in particular, as the beneficiaries of freedom, enjoying our rights, pursuing happiness while living within the bounds of truth and freedom. Fact triumphs over fiction. Science makes the best case. Inclusion works better than exclusion.

SOURCE: The Royal Society for the Encouragement of Arts, RSA, Article Title: Drugs: Facing Facts, March 2007
From the British publication, Daily Mail, March 9, 2007 page twelve article. The leading copy: Children of five "should be taught the danger of drugs" by j.slack@dailymail.co.uk & the Home Affairs Editor with another lead in headline: "Ecstasy is safer than alcohol" plus THE KEY CONCLUSIONS, an insert. Here are those conclusions as printed:

> DRUG laws not "fit for purpose" and need overhaul.
> USE of drugs should be 'regulated', not prohibited.
> A,B,C, classification system should be scrapped in favor of harm index.
> ALCOHOL and tobacco should be rated more harmful than Cannabis and Ecstasy.
> POLICE should focus on criminal gangs - and leave casual users alone.
> HEROIN should be prescribed to addicts to cut crime and "shooting galleries" introduced for users.
> DRUG education should begin in primary school.
> PRISON should be used only for those involved {distribution wise} with most harmful Drugs.
> ADDICTS should be protected from the sack if "managing" their condition.
> DRUG testing of crime suspects should be scrapped.

SOURCE: RSA: Drugs: Facing Facts, March 2007
Those(the above)conclusions are from the report done by The Royal Society for the Encouragement of Arts, Manufacturers and Commerce aka the RSA. It's English.

This report places Heroin at the top end of the harm scale, along with Cocaine, Barbiturates, and Street Methadone. Number five is Alcohol. After those first five come Ketamine, a horse tranquilizer, and (two) Amphetamines. Tobacco is ranked ninth, making alcohol and tobacco ahead of Solvents, LSD, the date rape drug GHB, & Ecstasy. Cannabis is ranked eleventh. <u>The report was produced by the RSA Commission on Illegal Drugs, set up in January 2005. The report also says:</u>

"The use of illegal drugs is by no means always harmful any more than alcohol is always harmful. The evidence is that the majority of people who use drugs are able to use them without harming themselves or others."

LaDeDa LaDeDa LaDeDa

Drug court is cheaper for the alleged felon but prevents the otherwise obvious revelation that individuals there are caught in a round robin of half truths and unconstitutional actions being used against them.

Loss of Liberty. We taxpayers are literally supporting our own oppression. With truth suppressed, lies repeated, our criminal justice system routinely makes fodder out of normal people who are run through punitive steps, often ending in incarceration, total loss of Liberty. All this is costly and dehumonizing to the non criminal and their families.

To so called constitutionally discriminate against the so called illegal drug possession people by treating them, us as the public, as outlaws legally requires another amendment to the constitution stating such. Accepting incarceration discrimination means accepting this scourge. Drug abuse of all sorts affects both users and non-users, all Americans and all the people of the world. This scourge still takes place due to the manipulation of our government policies by nefarious big money interests that rule us. The result is actual humon beings being criminalized for substances that ultimately and immediately are best regulated for best results. Anything else is not legal, not constitutional, and thusly becomes a Humon Civil Rights Violation of the first order.

Many institutionalized industries support enforcement of our nefarious laws or policies, such as The Law Enforcement Plutocracy: The Courts, Rehabilitation, Incarceration, Lab Tests for Urine Drug Detection, and on and on. All these industries are as deeply dependent as the pusher on the street on the contraband final consumer. That is bad well beyond the questionable good of employing people for the endless persecutions.

Treatment, Non Punitive Rehabilitation, Help, Compassion and Understanding work wonders, no doubt. Caring does not include tax payer supported punishment(s). Let us work to include everyone and everybody as in our care and do so without trespassing on Humon Civil Rights.

So many work to turn non criminal individuals, once convicted, into the fodder of a difficult so called criminal justice system. A difficult system impossible to improve or cease even as it systematically fails to benefit the public.

We The People Deserve Better! Ultimately we are wrongly diminishing our resources of humon productivity by daily making many victims through the unconstitutional loss of liberty of individuals who are found possessing, buying, selling, growing, or trafficking, in public.

Perhaps one is found in private with a search warrant, signed by a judge. People are losing their liberty over an Herbal vegetation containing no toxins. Indeed, it is an asset to the humon condition, is Cannabis. Pot can not intoxicate. No toxins.

bbbbbbbbbbbbbbbbbbbbbbbbb

All manner of sea worthy vessels including Jet Skis are trafficking Marihuana to California shores. The arrests are up thirty seven percent from last year. Warrants to search Ski Dos result in Pot Busts. November 11, 2013. The only legal Pot in California is grown in California. No imports allowed. Underground Pot in California is selling briskly because of pricing.

The natives are restless. Californians are chomping for their Creation Given Natural Resource Health Restorative and Superior Libation that is an asset to the humon condition as well as environmentally advantageous, Marijuana.

More than one million Americans were arrested on Cannabis related charges in 2011, alone, as victims of the law against what is intrinsically legal Marihuana possession. Arrests continue.

August 2013 our Attorney General, Eric Holder, is spear heading the conversation to revisit prison sentencing. The mandatory minimums are under scrutiny. Judges may be allowed to judge defendants as individuals again. A backdoor potential improvement change to a monster front door issue.

Investigation results show the ills of our judicial system stem from policy. POLICY. Memos and innuendo. Precedent. Once held up to the light we see the gaping holes where justice should be. Imagine.

~~~~~~~~~~~~~~~~~~~~~~~~~~~~~~~~~~

What has happened to truth and justice?

What does it cost American taxpayers to keep enforcing this so called 'law' against Marihuana possession for distribution? A Trillion Dollars every decade? Who knows?

It appears The Drug Abuse Prevention and Control Act of 1970 law as written never meant to criminalize Pot Heads.

Evolve the 'drug' laws implementation policy or stay surrendered to validating the enthronement of crime as organized crime, our permanent self induced self replicating foe. We the people lose, organized crime wins.

To close the circle, it is also true that ingesting, having ingested, even heavy recent reeking ingestion, is not illegal. Could get you some stares at the grocery store, or a frisking search for a gun on a New York City sidewalk, a procedure in place ten years. [This ruled as an unacceptable police duty by a judge much to Mayor Bloomberg's chagrin, August, 2013.]

What happens to a person with a Pot odor in public depends on factors like, where are you, who is there, anything and everything.

Pot in your body will cost you your employment if you flunk a drug pee test. Usually it's a pass/fail test for THC and other Schedule I classified drugs in the urine you provide by peeing in a cup with an attendant somewhere nearby. Suspended liberty, invasion of one's privacy, it's coercion to self incriminate at the very least.

No arrest for THC in pee for your Equal Opportunity Employment attempt. You lose if it's an advanced test in a state with a law saying at what level one is over the limit and driving so called impaired is involved. No employment if the test is at a job's application threshold. Equal Opportunity Employers always eliminate an applicant for the job if the 'drug' test pee test is failed.

No 'drug' test? One possesses in private? Purchase and imbibe on private property, where no one cares about a little Pot aroma. In your castle, your home, you are not a criminal over the personal supply of Pot in your possession until the cops find it accidentally in person or you have a brush with law enforcement risking all to be revealed.

Over time the law bleed over to simple Pot possession in public as felonious. Policy. Largely a misdemeanor amount is under fifteen grams. An ounce of Pot is twenty eight grams.

-OOOOOOOOOOOOOOOO-

The following event took place Spring 1971, Central Park, New York City:

Four young people in their early twenties are sitting on a grassy knoll in Central Park, one warm early spring day with sunshine. They are passing a joint. Two plain clothes Cops approach from behind. Badges flash just inches away in front of two pairs of eyes.

Busted! The four ride in an old style delivery truck style paddy wagon to the police station with their captors. The plain clothes arresting officers apologize saying, "We're working in the Park as a punishment today. We popped you guys to end this duty, sorry."

Such was the broadly held notion of imminent legality for Pot. Spring, 1971.

The four are booked and come back for arraignment represented by Fox TV's own Geraldo Rivera, then a newly minted lawyer, same mustache and hair, decades away from silver. The judge fined the person who possessed four ounces individually bagged carried on his person as brought into Central Park to sell, the person with a rolled joint in a shirt front pocket, and the individual caught pinching the half smoked joint in their fingers. Each received a fine of twenty five dollars. The fourth person, exhaling smoke, case dismissed.

That was then, this is now. A steady drumbeat of demonization, no new scientific findings allowed, has meant no end to the ideological only debate over Pot legalization.

Policy rules. Draconian principles prevail. Truth is smothered year end, year out.

Until now. Now oxygen is coming into the normalization of tolerance of all sorts, like gays may marry. Tolerance is more fun and less expensive for taxpayers. Besides, who isn't War weary?

Without legal legitimacy we see Law Enforcement before The Supreme Court seeking the right to bring sniffer dogs right up to a home's front door doorknob so the dog may alert for narcotics. Car door handles in public places are fair game and account for many arrests. Dogs don't differentiate. They are trained to sniff for all narcotics, not one or another. Marijuana is being phased out of their repertoire where appropriate. Old dogs remain unchanged.

Case in point: Since Recreational Pot legalization is underway Narc dogs in Washington State are being trained to alert on illegal drugs. Pot is legal, so not Pot.

In Greece many dogs live openly on the streets. They are protected and cared for by the authorities. Each is trained to alert for 'drugs' or whatever, say a bomb. Go to the Acropolis and see several good size dogs lounging about happily as you approach the attraction. April 2010.

Ittttitttttittttittttittttittttti

It's the wrong time for more persecution. No ruling has come back from the Supreme Court on the residential 'drug' sniffing dog's legality. It's been many months. No ruling is the right answer. March, 2014.

uouuoouuouupuouuouuouuouu

Terry Gross did a National Public Radio interview that took place a week before the August 11th, 2013 airing on WGCU. She opened the interview saying that Baltimore is known as the worst American city for drug issues in the early seventies when cities had whole communities under siege by criminals. She is chronicling the history of the 'drug' war. As heard on WGCU, Ft. Myers, Florida, Terry asked the retired policeman about those days.

The ex Baltimore Maryland policeman spoke remembering and explaining why his cohorts and he in their day concentrated their arrest efforts in minority communities.

Listeners heard as noted:

"The folks in gated communities and such would be on the phone using their power and influence to protect their rights and privacy if we went into their communities. Besides we were pressured for volume of arrests and the minority communities were easy pickings, targeted. We could take our dogs out on the street to find the car door handles with a contraband scent the dog could detect." Early seventies.

all6s&7s6s&7s6s&7s6s&7s6s&7s6s&7s6s&7salla

Police arbitrarily approaching us in our homes on a door to door basis would ruin the respect given the place one lives as sacrosanct. A court ordered arrest warrant or search warrant has to be in hand to gain entry. A dog sits?

Please. To get a warrant there needs to be sufficient evidence to convince a judge that a law that actually serves and protects needs enforcement meaning there is reason to believe a conviction will be the outcome.

The final consumer of Pot is using out of the public sphere, rarely a criminal offense, yet is necessarily the biggest Pot consumer population numerically. The sniffer-dog-on-our-door-step proposal NOT being in place boils down to our police and sheriffs persecuting us within commercial arrests. In effect by merely blocking the door to legal sales law enforcement is literally fronting, shilling, for the self perpetuating lucrative underworld market. A hugely lucrative 'drug' business that is unregulated and concentrates monster tax free wealth into the hands of criminals, of every affiliation.

With Potheads there are too many of us to make the cut as criminal, budget wise. Never mind, Potheads like an asset not a detriment. Good People Like Pot.

Territories for selling 'drugs' become violently fought over by gangs and organized crime thugs. Innocent victims take bullets too often. Street battles are no longer in the news. Drugs are more sophisticatedly moved and sold, away from detection. Now the wars for territory are outside of the United States. Plus, due to economic hardship public funding for local Drug Warring is vastly diminished.

January 16, 2013 the Mexican state of Michoacan is in the midst of ousting the drug cartel, Knights of Templar, plaguing them since the War against the Mexican drug lords began in 2006. This is an actual battle taking place to displace the drug business infighting from inside to outside of their city. Only the conflict is dissolving into a three to four way fight, the federal government is fighting armed vigilantes, who believe the government is helping the cartel with help flowing to the vigilantes from rival cartels. It's a big wasteful mess, normalcy disrupted for everyone.

Even so the truth is ripe to be heard. Inclusion, not exclusion.

We the people want final consumer consumption protections per source and quality. We want safety of acquisition, cultivation and use of Cannabis. Like Uruguay is implementing.

Cooled smoke, edible Pot laced goodies, the better health, normal camaraderie, Yes. No more taxpayer supported imposed stress and incarceration as currently imposed on multitudes of Americans.

Pot Freedom could mean lower health care costs. The list of benefits available for humonkind make Pot a marvel. Why not awareness and change? Put the onus on our currently do nothing Congress? Forget it. The good news: The Judicial Branch and the Whitehouse are teaming up. Do we dare hope?

Late 2013, Eric Holder is mounting a serious release of prisoners whose mandatory sentencing has expired in it's excessiveness. First will come better transition services.

The yoke of evil suppression is creaking to a lifting off. That lifting off is an event preceded by We the People speaking out endorsing an America that lives Liberty and Justice for All. Spend for a Prison Inmate Assessment Program along with Just Laws. We will become a civilized people.

Suppose we think of our Federal Government as a Benevolent Despot. Noticing that the good people of twenty states and the District of Columbia have, most of them with petitioned induced referendums have, out of their own initiatives, started allowing prescriptions for Marihuana to be given and filled with astonishing results in demand with no statistical down side making the news. Noticing that allowing legal possession of Marihuana has no negative side effects for the user or non users, our benevolent Government being benevolent announces the suspension of all enforcement efforts pending a two year study for a possibly final determination. Such a sensible dream.

Partial dream come true. The Feds are to adhere to state Pot laws enforcement wise. Big Hip Hip Hooray. Late August, 2013 announcement by President Obama.

JjJjJjJjJjJjJjJjJjJj

Other older good news, April, 2013, President Barrack Obama steps up to create a Brain Initiative Study. Could that study verify that THC has receptors built in for THC in American brains too? Let us hope. THC is the active ingredient in Cannabis.

Many bad laws are still on the books, offenders untouched because the law has no place in modern times. For example, cohabitation is unlawful: un-marrieds living together as man and wife was punishable in one state in New England not so long ago. 2013 to be exact. Bad law can sit un-enforced on the books long before it's removed. Early 2013 the state legislature of Virginia took such a law off the books.

Remember what we Americans learn in civics class of those fortunate born Americans lucky enough to receive education in American citizenship. Every American has the duty and the right to stand up against tyranny. We each have the right to question and to have any law held up to scrutiny for constitutional legitimacy in the courts. The biggest tenet:

We hold each other accountable to do no harm to each other no matter what directive is given by whomever. Civilians, all Americans, can't be forced to do any acts against their will, legally.

Still every day law enforcement earns a paycheck illegally gathering for arrest the humon fodder to perpetuate the myth of narcotic drug possession as a threat to the public. The facts of harm done by narcotics possession and/or use simply do not support the criminalization that only perpetuates and grows the population of users exponentially.

The crime is the contraband market existing selling substances or activities without legal protections for the public and the vendor in place. There is a complete lack of benefit in this discrimination for the taxpaying public. Continuing the persecution of innocent people because we the public are brainwashed to go along with the program is no reason to further deny ourselves the opportunity to get to the other side of this scourge by experiencing no longer making contraband that which the consuming public has determined it wants. The public deserves to be served for the best outcome as common and practical knowledge direct.

Any and all behavioral crimes that are hurtful to our citizenry are illegal for everybody already, Cannabis possessors too. No added protections are gained by the public from systematic persecution for Cannabis possession. Instead, a magnitude and abundance of harm to all manner of citizenry worldwide is ensuing.

Occasionally the Drug War in Mexico is in the headlines. We bust significant cartel bosses giving the always fleeting appearance of resolving the drug war problems. Immigration and illegal border crossing has faded into a fight for the Hispanic and Latino(a) vote. Immigration reform predicated on a secure border between Mexico and the United States is no more than a tactic to never reform immigration law.

2014's midterm election begins the courtship for the Latino-Latina vote.

~~~~~~~~~~~~~~~~~~~~~~~~~~~~~~~~~~~

The 501(C)4 corporations are the anonymous donor big spenders for television advertising. Some few billionaires did their best to make a difference in the minds of the 2012 electorate. This is new. The Supreme Court ruled in 2010 that corporations are virtually people. Thus they opened the door to untold wealth using media shamelessly to sway the public with absolutely no one accountable. Negative ads appeal to conservative anonymous donor big spenders. Reporters have uncovered the several who are the richest givers to be staunch extreme right conservatives. The Koch Brothers, for example. In truth, we can not know what anyone personally believes, only what they pay for.

~~~~~~~~~~~~~~~~~~~~~~~~~~~~~~~~~

Contraband movers and shakers are made super wealthy tax free while placing extraordinary strain on tax payers to fight back. We as individuals pay for that desired health restoring vegetation, in the case of Marihuana. Worse than a conundrum. Some may believe that the users and the tax payers are mutually exclusive groups. Not so. Not even a little bit.

54545454545454545454545454545

Setting aside the pharmaceutical empire's designs on our money why not try natural choices. Throw your Pot seeds out the back door. We need freely home grown Marijuana as our first choice Health Restorative. Denying us this is serious oppression, persecution. Some suffer oppression, others loss of liberty, both are persecution.

We are prevented from living free of unwarranted persecution by use of the unwarranted power and control of our lives by law enforcement. The people of the world getting past this nonsensical anti loving one another hypocrisy is inevitable. Why not move ahead and start reaping the benefits of applying truth and justice now? Let the victimized and discriminated against live free.

Here is the story of an obviously legitimate beneficiary to be of legal Medical Marijuana residing in Florida as told in local news April 2014 on National Public Radio out of Tampa's University of South Florida Station:

A neighbor called in the fact that their neighbor has Marijuana plants growing in the backyard, was it four plants?

Two undercover cops arrive wearing ski type masks to disguise themselves from recognition followed by a SWAT team that didn't actually draw their guns, merely keeping their hands poised on their weapons. Bottom line the Florida State Attorney's office decided against filing charges. 2014 is a rough year to hide persecution. So Good Decision. Voting for legalized Medical Marihuana takes place in Florida November, 2014.

Our scientific community is blocked from scientific research on Marihuana. The facts we have about it's receptors in our brains, the placenta not passing Marihuana's THC to the unborn, the commonly known positive applications, all date from before the Narcotics Tax Act of 1937, or, were proven in another country. Marihuana largely remains out of normal scientific study reach in the United States. Who knows what fantastic use is yet to be discovered.

~~~~~~~~~

"We Potheads are not dysfunctional, much less criminal people. Cannabis is a proven asset to the humon condition. That puts the law on our side." -MKH

~~~~~~~~~

To arrest people, and/or confiscate THC providing vegetation, i.e. Cannabis possessing, cultivating, buying or selling, that arresting person(s)is, it appears, is subject to criminal prosecution for intruding or trespassing to separate a citizen from their personal liberty Without Just Cause.

Citizen arrests are valid. In what just court is there any defense for forcing Americans to buy illegally what is a known health aid with no negative side effects, that is, when left beyond the reach of punitive Marihuana law?

~~~~~~~~

"I assert my right to choose the remedy or recreation of my choice. Happiness pursued and found." -MKH

~~~~~~~~

Ask around. Try these truths in the courts. Acquire first hand knowledge. We want a world where it is okay to be okay.

Remember I'm Okay, You're Okay, the book? That was a sixties thing to help us get over the jitters in our post

World War II country. So much healthier, to maintain as our primary goal, health. War is inappropriate, 'Drug' or otherwise.

~~~~~~~~~

"We have seen the enemy and it is us." -Pogo

~~~~~~~~~~

Wake Up Call:

It is All of us. Now we see how interconnected we are by environment - One Planet, One Eco System, One Survival Location. We communicate. We are no longer allowed to persist stupid. Choose. Stop floundering around distracted by non issues. Time is of the essence.

Will we have enough Water? Affordable Good Water?
Will we have enough Food? Affordable Good Food?
Will Air stay Clean?
What about Renewable Clean Energy?

Are our children of the future to see our same chances to dream and build and grow more erudite and refined and knowledgeable or be stuck merely eking along in the mire?

We deserve better than to have the innocent bullied, abused, incarcerated, and damaged by our own government. When it comes to understanding the facts supporting legal use and the peoples' clear declarations for same we are ignored.

This must change, a change to believe in no matter which ideology you may defend.

Progress is being made by the Justice Department. Reform of mandatory sentencing is on the table. Early release of unfairly sentenced prisoners is forthcoming. State Marihuana law will trump the Federal law reference Pot, this administration anyway, it appears. Colorado and Washington State and now the city of Portland Oregon are legal for Recreational use and Taxation at the point of sale. At least Portland has taken a stand to this end.

Truth is persuasive once revealed.

~~~~~~~~~~~~~~~~~~~~~~~~~~~~~~~~~~

Could we simply stop paying for our persecution?

Legally, American tax paying citizens are allowed to withhold their tax money from the Internal Revenue Service, best in an interest bearing escrow account, while waiting for a probable trial to settle if the non payment has legal standing reference the stated reason, say the ill advised persecution of people favoring the use of Pot, and does so personally. If the finding is against the taxpayer the taxpayer pays up, with interest, no penalty. It is not against the law to disagree with the government and attempt a personal boycott.

Could this be so?

Tax reform is in the race to cross the bipartisan legislation finish line. Legal taxation boycotts would goose our Congressmun across the finish line to end boycotts. Yet the right to boycott government taxation is the very backbone of American individuality and freedom of expression. It's the peoples' one and only tool to really get the government to stop operating using false principles.

Such as shrinking government aid to our own people when more stimulus is needed to rev the economy. The middle class is under siege as well as the least of us. War is useless unless you are awash with government contracts for war related goods, like oil, petroleum, gasoline.

We learn December 2013 our economy is steadying up nicely and we won't wobble when the government stimulus large monthly dollars stop. We have an exiting Federal Reserve Chairman, Ben Bermanke. A woman, Janet Yellen, is to continue on in the Chairmon's post, 2014, affirmed November, 2013.

The eighty five billion monthly infused in the bond market by the Feds is recently dropped to seventy five Billion dollars a month as the weaning begins. We managed the Trillion dollar a year infusions in the American Bond Market every year for five consecutive years, 2009 to 2013's end. Banks use the infused money to trade in bonds without any risk of their own assets, meanwhile reaping the trades' profits. It's a sweet deal for our biggest banking institutions, still too big to fail.

!!!!!!!!!!!!!!!!!!!!!!!!!!!!!!!

"I advocate for legal Pot. I do not advocate anyone use Pot. I do advocate everyone have the choice." -MKH

!

Here is a direct response a person might do at the point of being the unlucky focus of a Pot bust, liberty lost.

Make a citizen's arrest charging the law enforcement individual who has charged you with a Pot crime the suspect. A suspect, badge wearing, citizen charged with a Humon Rights Violation while acting as a public servant. You may not be denied your constitutionally protected right against government intrusion without a Just Cause. No loss of liberty without a Just Cause. Serving and protecting means serving and protecting. We are not cloaked terrorists or assailants.

Illegally illegal Contraband does not define a person in the eyes of the law any more than education or religion. Money. Money buys legal smartz and power. It's time to put the prosecution on trail.

Prove contraband laws have merit, because they don't.

Pot is easily proven beyond a shadow of a doubt as an asset to the Humon condition. Ignorance is no excuse. You, yourself are also easily proven a non criminal, right?

Your presence in the community is stable and consistent, no offenses, good driver, good health, pays taxes, no victims either. Unharmed and unharming. Even if caught between binges of shop lifting and car jacking with a lengthy arrest record showing time served, present existence looking tenuous. You would still not be guilty of a crime associated with any Cannabis proximity. No Just Cause.

There is No Just Cause for a Cannabis possession or transaction or cultivation to be prosecuted as criminal. Cannabis use and possession and Cannabis selling and growing are a legitimate part of a constitutional law abiding life. No discriminating appropriate here. Arrest the alcoholic whose treatment is paid by insurance. Arrest the cancer patient dying of tobacco use. Arrest yourself for all the evil done under the guise of service. Ignorance is no excuse.

You may say you uncover the desperate misfit whose new life in the criminal justice system is a step to betterment. Help does not parade and look and feel like punishment, a punishment that tags you as ripe for all manner of perpetual discrimination of job denial from would be employers.

No more. We may not swarm to the streets demanding our freedom instantly, but rest assured Humonities love of Humanity will triumph. Truth and Justice shall prevail.

We in America are all sharing in the good life, some a very meager share. Some living a grandeur beyond knowing unless you are there. But material stuff isn't it. Not before health. Let's put ourselves individually, as teams of people on jobs, in offices, in the voting booths, everywhere on a focus of financial health, emotional health and by calming ourselves, physical health. Forget Prozac or Zolof or whatever is in now. Let's share growth on the national level again by letting our representation see and hear how we want our growth to NOT be out of FEAR, i.e. walls, arms, embargos, cutting much needed programs for the hungry and least powerful, instead emphasizing TRUST in our mutual dependence to get us anywhere GREAT, meaning for the GOOD of ALL. Speak and Call out the Future you want. It's Mystical, and referenced in the Judeo-Christian Bible, Islamic teachings and those for Buddhists, Hindi speakers, Muslims, why, it's in the hearts and minds of us all. Preparing for goodness and greatness is in the enlightened teachings of all our ancestors.

Yes, it sounds alarmist to speak up for peace. Why fear spending the coin of action for peace? On the contrary, why is it important to have the material and monpower for two big 'confrontations' at the same time? The Presidential Republican candidate in 2008, Senator John McCain, 2012, wants that preparedness in place, he says. Maybe we should add a third war ready army, to be really safe?

So that's one for the war we are mincing up to (Iran? They must say no to nuclear capability) and one for retaliating when some enemy thinks we are weak and makes another war. We're ready. Of course, the Afghanistan War will be over by then. And if asked President Obama will say "all options regarding Iran are on the table" 2012 campaign. And on it goes. April, 2013, wide attention is given to the young North Korean Dictator and his upcoming planned missile launch test. It tanked.

Iran has agreed to talk about giving up their project-able nuclear capability, January 2014.

August 2013 the uprising in Egypt has backfired and for better or for worse the day was saved by the military. The world looks on. Elections are about a year away. Syria is consumed by a nasty civil war. We give half hearted aid to the revolutionaries. The country has dissolved into many clan like factions. What to do? The to be deposed dictator is hanging on and has kept his own supporters.

Millions are displaced from Syria. America has taken in about a hundred refugees so far, early 2014. This is changing, we are told.

Again the world watches without decisiveness or involvement. Neither has appeal to any other government including our own. The worry is the economics of trade. Embargos and sanctions, frozen assets, tend to botch trade up. This is a tough time to lead on a global scale.

ohyeahohyeahohyeahohyeahoh

A paradigm shift is and was in the making. Is, people are psychologically unifying for change in the Middle East, over the Arab Spring it's called. Was, the winners are yet to emerge from the impenetrable dust and smoke of the confrontations. An interim President rules Egypt.

The Moslem Brotherhood is officially dubbed illegal in Egypt. This is awkward at best.

Pakistan and Israeli dignitaries may sit in a room together this month, August 2013. May they thaw out enough to agree on something. They agreed to take time off before a later meeting to meet to possibly agree on something.

The Syrian dictator 'Assad' used chemical weapons against rebels. September 2013 we wait for diplomatic resolution. The Syrian leader says he will give up all Syria's chemical weapons to avoid a strafing of fired missiles as punishment that would destroy the chemical warfare goods where they are. Time is now inserted to stall or delete that warlike step whose unintended consequences loom large. Secretary of State John Kerry is getting a work out.

Known as the National Security Agency Leaker, Edward Snowden's release into Russia as a refugee has cost Russia's Putin face time with our President this month. No Summit talks between these two heads of states. Snowden is a controversial whistle blower who wants the people of the world to know the magnitude of the surveillances of everybody's, all Americans, digital, meaning email and personal phone communication, by the National Security Agency, the NSA. Snowden's goal of public debate over these privacy invasions is well met. This is why Snowden contacted three journalists with his evidence, Summer 2013.

Shocking revelations. Mega data is mined, here and abroad. Yet individuals are pinpointed. Terrorists make these surveillances a must we are told. We were spying on our European friends as in Germany's Chancellor Merkels's cell phone. A decidedly unpopular move as seen by those overseas.

Drones operated by individuals thousands of miles away have taken out, murdered, lots of our targeted enemy individuals successfully. Maybe some were innocent? Some American citizens. This former crescendo of revelation from a young private in the United States Army. He worked monitoring distant drones while in Texas, the far away drones routinely killing multiple people in Far Eastern war zones. The perpetrator of this Classified Information Leak released to Wikileaks highly classified information.

Bradley Manning, now Chelsea Manning, has been sentenced in a military court to thirty five years for making known to the American public the videos showing this repeated killing. The appeals will take about four years. Four hundred thousand is the number of individual Bradley leaked 'documents' in 2011. Bradley received a Conviction, a Verdict of Guilty, sentencing in September, 2013. He's appealing a thirty five year sentence.

Controversy is on the backburner as we accept the damage done by drone targeted kills. Our security is being enhanced, we are told.

Because the Afgan deciders won't make an agreeable deal to the American military over American security, possibly meaning immunity from Afgan law, our presence there may mean zero before long when we wanted to stick around with some assets to continue keeping the Taliban at bay. The personnel for those assets need security, without that. . . .

It's not tumultuous times for American conflicts. Lots of hot and wet weather. California and Colorado have too many mammoth fires. Then there's too much flooding. Hugely destructive storms and tornados are wrecking havoc too often all around the country. Extreme weather, referred to frequently as climate change, is solidifying as a permanent issue.

December 2013 the cold weather is making news from southern California thru the mid west. Imagine or experience a long run of days below freezing. Power outages happening as though in a losers game of Russian Roulette. Oranges are saved from freezing in California by using giant fans and heat.

Get a brush with elation when you survive to feel good again intermittently. Mid January 2014 the Governor of

California declares a state wide drought. They have fires and snow melt.

BCABCABCABCABCABCABCABCABCAB

Economically the middle class needs real resuscitation. The Sequestration that began March 1, 2013 has hurt our recovery by half or one and a half percent of the expected growth in the economy. There have been several big disasters with trains and planes relating back to humon error it appears.

Above paragraphs are a thumbnail sketch of our historical moment August to December, 2013. Pot is tipping toward acceptable. Our economy is growing sluggishly.

December update. Florida's Supreme Court is deliberating to decide the fate of the People's Proposed Amendment to legalize Pot for Doctors to prescribe Pot. The wording on the petition is under fire from Florida State Attorney General Pam Bondi. She wants the court to say the wording is misleading and may allow low level pain sufferers to obtain Pot. She apparently draws the line of exclusion to make menstrual cramps acceptable suffering, no medicinal Herb allowed.

The number of acceptable registered voter petitioners required to have the Medical Marijuana Proposition on the ballet in November 2014 is accomplished before the February 2014 deadline. Still waiting on the state Supreme Court ruling about the admissibility of the initial petition's wording. Several other petitions got busy too.

?!?!?!?!?!?!?!?!?!?!?

Let's overwhelm the noxious countries, the already nuked up: North Korea, India, the USA, Israel, the UK, France, etc. Oh wait, we like ourselves and all but one on the list......? We could emphasize proper disposal and neutralizing, of all our antiquated old nuclear leftovers formerly at the ready, tons and tons and tons of highly radioactive junk. Plus we keep our radioactive waste on site at nuclear plants. An acceptable solution for radioactive waste storage is still needed.

sensibleisbettersensibleisbetter

We wait to see how the Syrian crisis turns out. We hear Syria will join a no chemical weapons conference as a member in good standing.

All the many wonderful countries making up our world's people have an option. We'll make joining in look good. We'll be like, "What will you bring?" and establish a new global market for countries who are willing to tell us what steps they are taking to make their people a sounder healthier people. No harming behaviors. A government against it's people, could be admonished trade-wise.

The governments in the cooperating counties are distinguished because they focus on righting their own internal wrongs and are supportive of each other.

Each is held accountable to stay in good standing. There are trade perks. We establish an Exchange of stuff and ideas and people. Trade is our economic backbone and the time is now. Seize the moment. Fashion a beautiful foundation of quality like the United States Constitution and we'll forget those adolescent like, nasty non participants who are still afraid to join in on the peace and happiness. The Platform for agreement isn't set to homogenize cultures although it might. Perhaps the best of all our cultural individuality surviving. When has sharing as friends and for profit not been satisfying? Try it, You'll like it.

Money is based on faith. Our whole world's financial gizmo. What we so charmingly call our global economy, has at it's core only faith. Keep the faith. This means worry not to fit the thread through the needle but look to the gladness of your finished garments. Prudence in one's practices is the part of the yield of our endeavors that becomes prosperity.

War is wasteful. None more so than the 'Drug' War.

Take a chance people of the world, we can always revert if we don't pull off a nice quantum leap into a satisfactory future where fair dealings with no animosity rule.

It's always been apparent that there is plenty of natural disaster and illness and plenty of improvements to be made both here and abroad where we may focus our attention. Picture a world where we do not thrive on hatred. Believe that goodness and truth deserve to win. How do we get there from here? Focus. Agree. Plan. Implement. Celebrate.

~~~~~~~~~~~~~~~~~~~~~~~~~~~~~~~

Mon's inhumonity to mon as never ending is not the American way. {Formerly known as "Man's inhumanity to man." See a Note that follows} For all these decades we Americans have held ourselves up as a functional democracy decrying humon rights abuses elsewhere. We posture ourselves as exporters of the democratic way of life yet have in place as criminal what is not even worthy as a stigma.

Marihuana possession is a Federal crime. Allowing Marihuana possession to be the catalyst to damage by a crushing of the humon spirit, humon mind or somebody's very body and soul by imprisoning individuals without cause in the final analysis is not sustainable morally or financially. Yet here we are, lacking the conviction of our Christian and what not values, so many of us blind to the truth. No, we make mandatory satisfaction of our demand other countries mimic our deluded 'drug' warring. For 'make mandatory' read receive American money in some form of aid.

Let's try Freedom. If freedom doesn't work out for us after all, we'll fix it. Right now the most powerful people in too many regions and seats of power make their money in the illicit drug trade.

March 20, 2014 we hear of a shift in congressional thinking. The sensible sentencing and reduced recidivism ideas are topical. A Bill in Congress is shaping to let the 'drug' related convicted criminals out of jail or sentenced for less time over the need to reduce prison populations and accept that the current situation of filling prisons erroneously is Draconian, all wrong, at best.

This new call to action is based on awareness. "Fiscally and morally beneficial" states a congressman into a microphone. A chink of truth wedges into the brains of some United States congressional Legislators. Thank God and National Public Radio for bringing us a show revealing this potential step to correcting in some measure this ongoing inhumonity.

Some speak of the fiscal loss to the prison operators.

Prisons hold all manner of non criminals. The mentally ill, the impoverished, illegal immigrants, and the mentally challenged are routinely housed in prisons wrongly.

Mentioned is the fact that where states have released prisoner non violent criminals so far the crime rate has not gone up.

Worst of all our civil servant police and sheriffs are tasked with arresting as criminals the local normal people who imbibe, or grow, or sell on their own local scale. Truth is, theirs are the same rights as the shoe salesmon's or grocer's or any businesses customers. If the customers don't come the business will fail. What policemon who has their own secret stash or not, is not also harmed when a fellow citizen, perhaps under aged, is dropped into the system with only a slim chance of coming out as good as they were going in? It's wrong a God Given Natural Resource Health Restorative and Superior Libation considered good for so many is out of legitimate reach.

We are taught not to put temptation in another's way. Don't leave your purse open in a busy grocery store, wallet in sight, and not be partially culpable if the wallet disappears. By maintaining 'drug' contraband every American adolescent will likely see the bright bling of the 'drug' trade beckoning. May each not be vulnerable. But are we not each of us culpable for forcing the most lucrative career facing many vulnerable young adults to be the most dangerous? Being charged with a crime and convicted is more damaging than most any other event to an individual, generally speaking, barring a loved one's surprise death, parish the thought.

Contra banding 'drugs' harms people. Why penalize people for Marihuana possession at all, much less to be penalized worse than a thief or murderer. That's persecution. Persecution by any other name stinks just as much.

abcdefghijklmnopqrstuvwxyz

NOTE: The dropping of the letter a in humon and monkind makes these words all inclusive. The fem'ale gender no longer has to infer itself as included. We wemun would like each womon to know she is included in every reference to all monkind. Men agree to a man. It's called monning up, the all inclusive. Fem'ale is reconstituted to be pronounced Female, second e silent.

syzsyzsyzsyzsyzsyzsyzyzs

How do the insurance companies or any employer verify the implied impairment that prevents employment of those testing positive for Marihuana's THC in their urine? There is no verification of impairment. Testing positive for THC in your urine equals No Job. Every ad for employment saying Equal Opportunity Employer translates to mean take a pee test. This baseless loss of the right to employment is a fundamental infringement of every American's Civil Right, the right to lawful employment. Reads like a class action suit in the making, doesn't it? Also great for motivating entrepreneurs. Legislators could be moved to Act.

In the states with legal medical Marihuana, does the state's valid law legalizing prescription's as an exemption for use of Pot legally prevail and negate a prospective employer's insurance requirements for a so called clean urine 'drug' test result? Does a person in one of the medical Marihuana states not get charged with a DUI, Driving Under the Influence? After all the body holds on to THC for months, long past any so called 'altered state'.

Impairment is not codified officially as yet. Measuring the saturation percent of THC in urine is currently not in place. {Suggested numbers to follow.} Colorado is working on it. Impairment of any kind is against the law. We are charged with failure to have our vehicle in our control if that's the case. That's crime enough. No direct connect ensues by testing positive for THC. It's merely piling on. The RSA, Royal Society for the Encouragement of the Arts, with their well funded study say, "Stay away from testing urine" all together. The English RSA is the equivalent times two of America's Food and Drug Administration, the FDA. The RSA may well be more responsive as well.

syesysyesyesyesyesyesyesyesyesyes

Unlike the drug alcohol impairment, where alcohol content in the bloodstream is measurable by a breathalyzer, no such measurement exists for Marihuana.

Impairment from Cannabis is illusive, non existent. For the last ten years ten thousand people have lost their life on our roads every year because of a drunk driver, no change for the last ten years. This is preventable. Court ordered ignition control breathalyzers would help so much. Please note such a device may be purchased over the counter, late 2013.

Instead, Law Enforcement Officers are swabbing inside the mouth of a suspect, say an erratic driver. Is this an unlawful invasion and for what do they hunt in someone's inner cheek inside their mouth, THC? DNA?

Consider the coincidence factor. The momentary erratic driver is likely the temporarily distracted driver. Most folks perform as good or better drivers on Pot. Sleep depravation is the biggest culprit for driving failures.

Distractions are neck and neck. Cell phone conversations and texting are so dangerous when one is driving.

Pothead people don't knock down the cones on the course and may well have Safe Driver Designations on their Driver's Licenses. Marijuana does not depress the nervous system. No loss of judgment and/or coordination takes place. A Pot high is not the kind of intensity that poses a threat to the individual or others. That would be alcohol or nicotine as the lethal drug most harmful, abundant and ubiquitous.

No, there is no substantive argument to make against responsible adult Marijuana use. There is no way for others to even know if someone is 'high' unless they tell you or a physical manifestation is present like a residue of odor. Hardly criminal.

Imagine this controlled study: A number of individuals are invited to a faux party. The experiment is to discover if those questioned are able to correctly identify which people are high. This to discover if those questioned are able to determine which people are high on Pot from everyone else. Possible? Not likely.

A first time Pot user might be visibly moved at the enlarged perspective and greater concentration of focus, showing surprise at how much more known the moment may become. Unbiased science needs to weigh in with fresh new reliable data. Why would a pee test be necessary if there are observable objections to using Pot? Manifested deterrents. There are no known associated deterrents to possession and in reality, no law against use. This proves it is persecution to be relieved of one's liberty or employment opportunity over Marijuana in one's mouth or pee or possession.

Too bad scientists can't do Marihuana studies until it's legal. The FDA has roadblocks up. It seldom permit's a study. If one qualifies to do a study it must be with participants who are 'experienced users' and willing to live in a hospital for the duration. Now we know.

Here's a theory: The US Army made an opinion during the Korean War for President Eisenhower about Marihuana, and later for President Kennedy preceding the Vietnam War. Marihuana was seen as appealing to bright men who began to question, especially in Vietnam, the army's logic and their, the soldier's, vulnerability. Dangerous.

A soldier works for survival with his fellow soldiers as worthier than dying needlessly. This because they have enhanced thinking and have penetrated to the obvious, that if they don't take care of themselves they are dead meat. These are the men who protected each other with clever tactics. Ask a survivor of the fighting United States military in Vietnam.

The bottom line for all the persecution: Contraband sellers stay rich, and besides all the usual legitimate business opportunity perks created by persecution, persecution contributes mightily to a cheap labor force.

The unchallenged market share given the super rich provides a Cheap Labor Force, resulting in enhanced shareholder outcome. Currently we are experiencing a shift to much downward pressure on the Middle Class set in motion by the housing market collapse precipitated by mortgage manipulation, the escalated ripping off by Mortgage Securities bundling and selling on and on up the chain to ever more ridiculous worth. All this nefarious activity culminates at the potentially impending end of our country's and the world's economic stability. The United States Congress Republican House members allowed our collective necks to stretch hanging us out over the ledge dropping off to worldwide financial collapse up to a mid October 2013 deadline. Luckily, we may have real economic traction on the way, mid November, 2013. Although the noose is swinging empty it is handy, waiting for mid January 2014. Bad Tea Party, don't touch!

Congress managed to extend the debt ceiling raising and our country's collective well being to January 2015 passing American fiscal responsibility for a whole year, done January 2014.

Banks, we are told, are too big to fail. Government money, taxpayer funding, bails out the teetering over bastions of feckless economic security decisions. The middle class is the player left without a chair when the music stops.

+=+=+=+=+=+=+=+=+=+=+=+=+

The fear of those of us basically without political power becoming enhanced by a Weed has resulted in the politically powerful maintaining demonizing Cannabis and applying suppression. Unintended consequence? The walls put up backfire. It's a bonanza for criminals. Bootleggers, the mafias, cartels, pushers and home growers get busy. We are reaching the hundred years mark of supply being illicit for hard or the most addictive harmful drugs, that is, most harmful before lab drugs came along. The underworld suppliers provoked inflated demand for the hard or harmful addictive drugs. Persecution and prosecution for uncontrolled controlled substances became the daily norm.

March 2014 Boston's heroin addicted population is besieged by a killer poison laced heroin. The siege took thirteen lives? Perpetrator uncaught? Resolution unknown here.

Once Pot was criminalized and demonized erroneously the minorities took the brunt of persecution. The white world largely not targeted for persecution or prosecution until the seventies when additional thinning out of Baby Boomers became popular too with those satisfied status quo types unmoved by peace and love as possible market forces. That's when the local gangs got product to sell making them huge wealth and into stable powers. Gangs got busy. Thus was the creation of the carnage of territorial 'drug' wars. Gang wars cause many innocent people to suffer damage or death.

sdfsdfsdfsdfsdfsdfsdfsdfsdfsfds

Who experiences Potheads as a menace? A common put down or dishing on potheads is,

"What have you been smoking?" Said to someone who speaks about something in such a novel way the hearer dismisses the remark thusly.

A common remark about a known pothead, not present, "Joe's always busy and gets results." Ha Ha!

Media personalities do their mellowed out voices and speak of odd behaviors to convey stoned. That's a narrow part of the spectrum should it exist. Know the top oncologist in a renown California hospital who declared himself as an early in his life adherent to the intrinsic value of Marihuana. He is heard Fall 2012 speaking in a conversation on National Public Radio, with an NPR interviewer and a spokesmon for the Food and Drug Administration, the FDA, making a three way conversation. The oncologist was there to promote understanding of the good pot does the terminally ill with cancer as reason to provide genuine legality for their Pot.

Pot on mainstream television and in print continues to be marked as a target and no wonder, media money comes from the big corporations advertising dollars. Big business fails to see any advantage to unleashing a potent competitor. Present advertisers want to keep Pot illegal. Like everything, change is inevitable and big business is adapting even now.

For certainly the tide has turned.

Colorado and Washington state just voted yes to recreational Pot, up to one ounce in Colorado per adult person, legal as of January 1, 2014.

Legalization, no catches, is unexplored territory. The legality of growing and selling must be factored in with licensing. If the voting public make something true, whether bridge to be built, or Pot in the hand, the government has it's marching orders to perform, whether the government grows the Pot or licenses others to do so. The consuming public is paying tax to purchase legal Pot taxed at twenty six percent in Colorado early 2014.

Legalization generally begins at the point of the tally result certification unless a predetermined start date for implementation is stated within the newly approved law.

Opposition to truth is best seen as ugly. It's been said that Truth is Beauty. Not the groomed to perfection standard of a glossy magazine commercial photo shoot.........

Beauty,
The Natural
Honest
Creation
We
Maximize
As Our
Culture
Country
And
Selves

This is no time to be adversaries. All our government has the same boss across the board, all of us. Finding how to please us is the goal of government.

&&&&&&&&&&&&&&&&&&&&&&&&&&&

All medicine derives from plant matter. Vegetation, the elements, any and all earthly substances are the backbone of all medical science laboratory innovation as well as the entire history of exploration and development that makes up the lore of medicine and people since time. As one United States Congressman put it erroneously, to be a medicine Marijuana needs the approval of the FDA, the Food and Drug Agency in charge of what we get to purchase and consume. Their goal being properly marked products to tell the consumer what to expect taking a pill or eating a soup.

They don't approve apples or oranges. They don't label whiskey or gin. They need Congress to put the words Addictive Deadly Poison on Cigarette packs. No luck so far not for lack of trying.

Recent early February 2014 the Tobacco horror story is all over the media. Big health care issue. The bottom line: have our children decide not to ever try tobacco with education. Currently, for every person who dies of tobacco two people become smokers.

Circa 1959 seventh graders received six weeks of instruction about Tuberculosis. Thirteen year olds sat at their desks making their own brad held white blue lined hand written paper report in a blue report cover. The cover had a red logo also hand done.

Each student dutifully produced on their own paper the sketch of the Sputum, coughed up drops of blood, one of all the illustrations presented with all the necessary explanations. The idea was that knowing how TB is transmitted through the air, making holding your handkerchief over your nose and mouth on an elevator acceptable, a good way to prevent spread. There were department store elevators. No violent coughing took place.

Children are open to propaganda to keep them aware of potential pitfalls. Why not the Understanding Drugs Monual?

Maybe also known as U D Mon!?!

Pot is a naturally occurring vegetation with an ingredient our minds, bodies and souls are prepped to receive with exclusive receptors, THC. Pot enjoys five thousand years of appreciation in written and oral history. FDA approval? No, who would make it worth their while? God? Could be. No patent, no interest.

Switzerland allows a quantity of ten grams in an individual's possession of Marijuana as long as that person quietly accepts the equivalent of an American hundred ten dollar unrecorded 'misdemeanor' fine.

Here in America we have uncovered seventy five underground tunnels linking Mexico to San Diego Warehouses since 2008. This became news again in early February 2014. The story is the blighted life of an individual who was tricked by his captors into being a person digging a new such tunnel. This individual makes his plea for justice saying it's "the right thing" when interviewed while serving jail time in California for the digging in spite of being an abused slave of the actual criminals. Thus adding to the Systemic over crowding of jails with the innocent, mentally ill, and hard core incompetent.

A United States Congressman has called for hearings and has conducted the introduction. He has concluded that the government would do well to reconcile the riff between state and federal law regarding Cannabis. We shall see. He did mention NORML, The National Organization for the Reform of Marijuana Law at the end of his list of entities to appear for a grilling on the subject.

Historically Eric Holder announces February 11, 2014 the Federal Government will recognize all legal marriages, including single gender couples.

Humon beings would willingly be studied in legitimate documentary settings with their Cannabis to see the lawful ease of Pot acquisition openly enjoyed everywhere.

Throw out some seeds and nature does the rest. Soon whatever superior results of Cannabis, as consumed compared to patented dangerous side effect pills, could be widely known. The use of little pipes and rolled joints could be passé, replaced by cooled smoke and edibles. Inhalers for those preferring Cannabis Hi Tech. Or choose a modern Hookah, a water pipe with usually several limbs for inhaling.

The manufacturers of competing lab drug pills are one of the constant forces driving to keep up the criminalization of Pot use in public. Lawmakers abiding by the honored kings and queens in their castle, aka a sanctioned home front, as penetrable only with a search or arrest warrant. If you patent your land then you are sovereign. You may be naturally sovereign if you live in some parts of Texas.

Aside. Now we have the Patriot Act. That's a real belt tightener for freedom. Hello NSA, the National Security Agency intelligence gathering monster that our NSA Leaker Edward Snowden revealed as spying on us. Summer, 2013.

The NSA's intelligence gathering has been in place for years and all of us were and are subjects.

....

Demonizing Pot is the underlying conceit, a false premise. It blinds the public's eyes to the two headed monster that is illicitly feasting on the American public. One monster head, the providers of the contra banded drugs. The other? Our Local, State and Federal Law Enforcement empowered by an ignorant Congress in concert make the other monster head of the two headed monster.

Lately sale of Cannabis is said to be the big time money maker. Cannabis sales are carrying the overhead of the small time money losing demand for the traditional hard drugs of yesteryear, heroin, morphine, opium and cocaine. Australia is coming through a wave of massive cocaine popularity among there young upwardly mobile citizens, 2012. Opportunity abounds for the underworld because individuals in the underworld are expendable and replaced. When one goes down another steps up.

Even more lately, the push from pushers of heroin is helping heroin make a comeback on the back of the loss of easy to purchase pain killer mill pills.

Our plight is the drug contraband scourge is done the pusher's way. The resulting illegal drug damage to many is actually held in place by the illegality of having no regulation for consumer protections, something un-American. Criminalization of Cannabis leaves the entire population of growers, traffickers, buyers and sellers outside the umbrella of civil protections. That should be unthinkable in a free country whose people pledge Liberty and Justice for all.

These simple words make light of the hundred years since 1914. The American public has been harmed by this negative push me, pull me. Every turn of Congressional legislative history regarding what's contraband reveals the underlying Congressional legislators, elected individuals with the winning input, erred by bowing consistently to ignorance and petty and horrific greed, hypocrisy. We the people know short shift well, also known as The Shaft.

Internet search to read about The Harrison Narcotics Act of 1914, The Marihuana Tax Act of 1937, and Tetrahydrocannabinol.

Peruse the Supreme Last Word reference 'Drugs' in written law in about two hundred seventy pages; the Controlled Substance Abuse Prevention Act of 1970. It's Acts date forward to 2010 as of January 3, 2012. A list of the thirty six acts passed into law by the United States Congress from 1970 are an outline of the march of the lucrative American Drug Scourge. See pages 115 to 117, this book, for the list of thirty six Congressional Acts.

Enhancement with Pot equals an improved immune system as more oxygen reaches the brain and other organs from improved blood flow carrying more oxygen. Cannabis is the key to unlocking mental function upgrades causing subtle improvements in ability and perception both mentally and physically. Try your tennis game or an equivalent activity while high. You'll see.

Our moneyed powerful in government retaliate against increasing awareness of Pot's attributes. There is a Really Huge Money push to keep the oppression and the persecution 'legal'. A multi-tentacles empire informs who may be employed reference the pee test hurdle to employment, and who is subjected to persecution by arrest and what methods of persecution are employed. Check out the illicit drug sniffer dogs on our doorsteps legalization push heard by the Supreme Court now months and months ago. Still no ruling, late, 2013. Or March, 2014.

In national pole results announced in early April 2013 we the people are now at fifty two percent approval of legal Pot for all, not just the medically needy. Maybe the Supreme

Court is aware. Latest is fifty seven percent. More media personalities are jumping on board too.

Florida residents recently poled at eighty two and seventy six percent, respectively, approval of medical Marijuana, Democrats and Republicans. This the backdrop for a State Court to rule on the admissibility of the Proposition to Legalize Marihuana for Medicinal Use for the November 2014 ballot. The question is, does the wording mislead the public.

No! The vote for Medical Marihuana is proceeding to the ballot for the upcoming election in Florida November, 2014.

Republican by Definition - supporter of republic as government: somebody who believes that the best government is one in which supreme power is vested in an electorate.

{Encarta ® World English Dictionary © & (P) 1998-2004 Microsoft Corporation. All rights reserved}

Democrat by Definition - supporter of democracy: somebody who believes in democracy and the democratic system of government and argues in favor of them.

{Encarta ® World English Dictionary © & (P) 1998-2004 Microsoft Corporation. All rights reserved.}

What the federal government does in the well funded War on 'Drugs':

Congress creates committees and requests studies and reports and field work and experts and pays per-diems. All the legislation our Government bureaucracy passes causes dispersal of our tax payer money with each Act enacted by Congress as funding is built into every bill that passes.

Congress controls the purse string rules. Congress determines the funding for a falsely premised war. An Illicit

Drug War. Repeat. Repeat. Repeat. Still expecting other than the undesired results? Insanity by popular definition.

Now we know the initial inclusion of Marihuana in the Narcotics Tax Act of 1937 is unequivocally based on falsehoods paraded as truth. One man in government, Anslinger, as head of the Narcotics Bureau, crusaded with false anecdotal evidence. {Narcotics as Illegal Codified in 1914, thus a Narcotics Bureau in place,1937.}

Angslinger's highlighted coup de grace on truth:

A well documented deranged man who murdered, is passed off as a Pot induced homicidal maniac. A story similar to the one in the Reefer Madness genre movies of the era. More details to follow.

:X:X:X:X:X:X:X:X:X:X:X:X:

The humon effort surrounding the illicit DRUG WAR is staggering and costly to we taxpayers beyond our knowing. This ongoing oppression equals systematic dismantling of individual lives at apprehension and whole families at incarceration.

All individuals live in the pursuit of happiness. It's an inalienable right, "pursuit of happiness" is, as stated in the Preamble to the United States Constitution. No one, no government, can productively persist personal Liberty withheld.

Our reelected President Obama is hamstrung by the unyielding wall of resistance the Republican side of the aisle of Congress serves up as filibusters and hearings galore to make fake outrages center stage. Such gyrations are staged to obscure any Democratic efforts, in effect, draining momentum out of the Obama administration begun in January 2013. The Republicans are uncompromising with unmatched vengeance in presidential history.

By December 2013 Harry Reed took a vote on adopting as a Rule in the Senate, the so called nuclear option. A vote tally of a simple majority passes a bill. Fifty one votes, not the extra nine making the sixty formerly required.

Had to happen or the next three years of the Obama administration would be a bust. So much government business had halted by simply lacking Congressional approval that Senate House Majority Leader Harry Reed had no choice. We need governance to proceed with judges and other appointees put in place. And there will be more legislation we like if we are lucky.

The sequestration pain kicked in March 1,2013. Yet, things are somewhat changing for the better. We are mixed. It's early, May 19, 2013.

Flashback: the November 2012 election, January 1, 2013. We faced a seriously compressed amount of time to see our United States Congress make decisions on a list of seriously challenging Legislative must decides. At the top of the list is the sequestration issue, the variable cuts, across the board at percentages of 5% to 8.2% funding lost. Reductions in funding set to hit the Entire Defense Department including the Pentagon and every Federally funded anything with exclusions like Social Security and soldier pay checks.

We watched Congress jump up and perform in an instant over the furloughing of our nationwide Air Traffic Controllers, per the sequestration cuts, once the flying public had massive delay inconvenience one fine Monday in April 2013. That outrage lit into Congress and money was found to fix this issue and make an instant law, passed and implemented, that very week.

The food programs and assistance programs need to find a way to handle their funding reduction.

Another real upset is the automatic laying off of a million of our Federal employees from soldiers to Federal offices personnel.

This pain no gain occurrence is the direct result of the 112th United States Congresses' failure to agree. It came down to a standoff in Congress. Republicans refusing to give up extending the Bush tax cuts for the wealthiest, Democrats demanding the tax cuts remain for the middle class but not the wealthiest. We already lost our AAA credit rating to tarnish over the protracted time The Tea Partiers in Congress took refusing to raise the debt ceiling. Congress controls our nation's purse strings and the debt ceiling needs to cover allocated spent money to be paid, not future spending. Yet there is no compromising. We are in a partisan gridlock.

Same story, different day. Congress did fund to the twenty eighth of September 2013, as the new projected end of existing funding to pay the government's bills. Eight days away from the twenty eighth of September the public's future was tossed about on the seas of Drastic Threats. Why not shut down the government? the Tea Party Republicans ask. Easy to say, hard to do. We pray.

The 2012 gridlock extraordinaire in Congress created the bipartisan, six of each, Republicans and Democrats, twelve person committee. The impasse had been too much for Congress. No vote passed in the House and Senate over the budget. And then No Budget from the committee of twelve. Only problem, the committee had the Sequestration Sword of Damocles hanging over it. Perform by deadline, i.e., agree to what and how much to cut who, or else on March 1, 2013 we all watch across the board cuts sweep across nearly all the Federally funded. The individuals to be affected unidentified. Expectations run high the Mandatory Sequestrations, or going over "The Fiscal Cliff", will not happen.

Note: We are AAA again, mid August 2013. The cuts are cut. The pain is felt. One consequence alone is fifty seven thousand Head Start Program children are now left unfed, school year 2013 to 2014. Turns out private resources stepped in to pay for the unfunded food.

Pre January 1, 2013 Congress could have solved the problem by backing off the cliff of sequestration in a post election, pre inauguration Lame Duck Congressional vote.

Because the 113th Congress is running fiscally with a budget that cannot add to the deficit the cuts are required. This per the Norquest Pledge the Republican Tea Party Congress people signed.

The mid term elections of 2010 swept into Congress the ultra fiscally Conservative Republican Tea Party people now dominating the Republican controlled House of Representatives. Our Congress is our government's purse strings, allocating all the funding and is responsible for making up the country's budget.

Mid December 2013 John Boehner has begun to make the noises of a ticked off House majority leader. The less truculent Republicans are realizing that the schism in their ranks is likely to bring them down from the voting booth. The ultra fiscally conservative Tea Partiers are not people conscious. They like big business to have big profits and little overhead. The Economic stability of Americans is less to them than an intangible number change in the deficit to smaller.

Consider all this upset over government spending is a screen hiding the devastating fallout to our country of the Republican George W. Bush presidency that took a President Clinton balanced budget, no debt, no deficit, to two trillion dollars in the red.

Go back to 9/11/02, the day of the terrorist attack on New York City's World Trade Center. When the Twin Tower buildings fell and three thousand people died we watched pitifully helpless, left only to mourn those who died in the devastation. Pause to reflect.

We created the Homeland Security expense, plus two wars, Iraq and Afghanistan. No thought to curtailing big spending. Like the story goes, "a billion here and a billion there, pretty soon you're talking big money." Anonymous.

Unprecedented spending.

The pendulum swings.

Along side the new Homeland Security expense, we started a War in Iraq. We got rid of Sodom Hussein, statue and dictator. Sodom was found hunkered down in a one man crevice covered in dirt, it was reported. He was quickly dispatched to his maker.

Poor Iraq remains in shambles politically and literally and we are basically out of there. We are helping financially still. March, 2014.

Next began the chasing down of Alquida terrorists on the impossible terrain of Afghanistan leaving the Alquida boss man, Osama Bin Laden, to hide in the mountains in a secluded cave.

The 110th Congress deregulated Wall Street. Thus the subsequent crisis of 2008 brought on by George W. Bush's and Clinton's deregulation of the lending industry. Deregulation removed oversight supervision of hedge funds and the like. The American housing industry went to it's knees because we gave carte blanche to Wall Street money manipulators. Home Loans were bundled and resold and resold for more and more.

With volumes of bad loans, no collateral or ability to pay, and obviously bad borrowers being approved for loans, loans began failing, borrowers not paying one by one. Home values took a dive and gave birth to the massive numbers of short sales and foreclosures not yet faded over the horizon in many markets, March 2014. Burst Bubble. A bubble pumped up with greed top to bottom.

January 2009 to March 2014, the years of watching the Bush Great Recession leave the headlines to seeing American governance itself so disrespected we are still in the shallows of recovery across our country. Big Money currently looking to buy the Republicans a bigger berth in Congress to further their no additional education or infrastructure money for the people after the 2014 midterm elections.

The electorate must make themselves penetrate the scope of the Republican Scheme of perpetuating the status quo that persists oppressing all but the wealthiest people. The Republican game plan is to Win Elections by flooding the media with their propaganda of emotional half truths and smear campaigning with no agenda of governance offered.

OOOOOOOOOOOOOOOOOOOOOOOOOOOOOO

Post Script: Osama Bin Laden is dead. President Obama ordered the attack during his first administration. Bin Laden was hiding in his compound in Pakistan. A United States Army Special Ops team quietly went into Pakistan, found Osama and shot him dead. Good sleuthing.

*4*4*4*4*4*4*4*4*4*4*4*

Ah, greed.

A short cut analogy: Our shiny ship of state is taken on a wild ride ending one fine fall day in the year twenty zero eight. Our ship ends broken apart into pieces on rocky shoals. The Captain, George W. Bush. His administration and the world's banking top echelon fully enriched, scramble away unscathed.

Bankers in league with those top bankers, found in London, England, we are told, get handed bailout money. The bailout passed the 111th Congress in the last quarter of 2008.

The helm for the totaled ship of state, our economy, is then summarily handed over to the newly elected President Obama, January 6, 2009. When the dust settles the American people have given billions upon billions of dollars in bail outs to the banks and the American automobile industry. The banks being too big to fail, and all. President Obama bets on the future success of the American Automobile Industry. He won that bet, by the way.

Note: Banks have generally returned their bail out money, too.

The Federal Reserve Chair Ben Bernanke had his last press Conference December 18th, 2013 for over an hour. The eighty five billion dollars the Federal Reserve has spent to purchase bonds, eighty five billion a month every month for several years now, is beginning to be tapered off. The stock market took it well. It's believed the money kept inflation and interest rates down for Americans. The new Federal Reserve chair Yellen, a woman, will preside much as Bernanke has, we are told.

The math: $85,000,000,000, eighty five Billion dollars a month, is twelve times $85,000,000,000 or $1,020,000,000,000. This is over one Trillion Dollars a year!

It sure does cost us a lot to stay rich or poor as the case may be.

Imagine if a Trillion Dollars a year had been spread across our population for the last five years. What a real stimulus to the economy. Each and every American, let us say we are about three hundred fifty million People. It works out to about three thousand dollars, $3,000, a year for everyone, all ages, all family members. Way cool. Could we find ourselves in paradise economically? The poor no longer too poor? Imagine a family of five with an added fifteen thousand dollars for five years. Transforming. Then we would be weaned slowly off the money with more money for a time, quantitative easing, it's called.

Perhaps it's a flawed plan. Think of the all important investors owning bonds. They are not just individuals. Bonds might remain strong in the face of so much money changing hands. Too late now anyway. The stimulus money is set to dwindle down, from eighty five Billion to seventy five Billion, as we the public are hearing the numbers in the media for the first time as we learn the Federal Reserve stimulus details,

The National Debt made news October 2013 by surging $328 Billion, three hundred twenty eight Billion Dollars. A surge of three hundred twenty eight Billion dollars took our National Debt to over seventeen Trillion Dollars for the first time.

Are the five years at one Trillion Dollars per year for the last five years, Five Trillion Dollars of Federal Reserve Money as Stimulus Dollars, included in the National Debt number of seventeen Trillion Dollars? Each Trillion dollars is one thousand of Billions.

No, the eighty five billion dollars government stimulus money monthly is 'committed' to buy government bonds and mortgage backed securities. Banks then say we'll buy those for you. So the government then puts the eighty five Billion Dollars stimulus money into the banks' various Reserve Accounts at the Federal Reserve. The banks are making unreserved money selling and trading those bonds and mortgage securities. The money in their Federal Reserve accounts is available like a bank account to them and they keep the profits.

The plan as presented to we the people was meant as a stimulus for banks to increase loans to Americans to create actual stimulation of the economy. Evidently the banks feel more like sitting on the funds, the bar to borrow is set too high or we are too hammered down in the aftermath of the Great Recession to be acceptable borrowers. Likely all three.

boohooboohooboohooboohooboo

2012, Americans are still questioning the whereabouts of the help as mortgage defrauded individuals and those caught in the failed housing market were promised. House by house values sank well below the homeowner's mortgagor appraised mortgaged homes' current dollar value. Their home purchase price or refinance loan is well over market value for their home. Their property is said to be 'under water'. Some people lost real cash paid to purchase their home, some gained free housing for years in no equity mortgages.

Some benefit is gained from reasonable refinancing with dropped interest rates. Programs exist that are under utilized. The Great Recession, first felt late 2006, is behind us officially since 2009.

We are five years past the Great Recession named in 2008. We are in the middle class blues period, end of 2013. Growth is in place. Good numbers are up, bad numbers are down. Only the economy is lackluster reference Holiday consumer purchasing. Year end sales money retailers are dependent upon may not materialize. [They did all right.]

The Federal Reserve Chair changes hands January first. Tapering off the monthly infusions of Federal money buying bonds is beginning 2014. March 2014 there's talk of interest rates going up. The historic thirty year low of an average three and a half percent is up to about four and a half.

For sure money in a bank account or Certificate of Deposit has earned practically zilch for a decade. Interest paid on saved money had been a way middle class folk gained monetary assets. You could let the interest roll over for years and see real profit from a modest investment in saving.

This worked well to pass on increased wealth to the next generations thus making the middle class more powerful. College tuitions were not borrowed. Illnesses didn't put families in bankruptcy. The middle class thrived.

soooooooooooooooooooothereeeeeeeeeeeeeeeeeeee

Where are the indictments for the criminal actions behind the housing debacle that made a debacle of our economy? Not one indictment has taken any of the known really top individuals who pushed such universally damaging greed. Meaning the London banker mini cartel to be exact. Actually not one person at the tip top has been indicted.

One indictment of a top managing hedge funder is Arthur G. Nadel. He was a top hedge fund manager who died in a North Carolina correctional institution, age eighty, 2012, a nice size fish. Just not one of the big killer whale size sharks.

Def>tdeftdeftde<fidgeted*ftdeftdeft!deftd

Lending is now the exact opposite of lending during the Big Run Up to Bust times. "Fog a mirror get a loan," Realtors jokingly said referring to placing a mirror beneath a person's nostrils to check for life. Stated income, no income verification, no problem. There was much real honest to

God, mortgage fraud and forgery, robo-signing even. Robo signing is the term dubbed to describe an individual that sat affixing fake signatures to lender to borrower contracts as their constant job.

After the Bursting of the Housing Bubble lenders demand 1)twenty percent down payment minimums, 2) a verifiable good income stream, 3)a credit score of about seven hundred and sixty, as a minimum 2013. Loaning is a cleaner version of the old ways with borrower scrutiny an initial high hurdle. It's grueling to borrowers forced to document their lives for the last twenty years, in some cases. That is improving with time.

Interest rates went to an all time low, under four percent, touching briefly down to three percent. September, 2013, there's a plateau again four to five percent. Banks borrowing at zero percent, still, February 28, 2014.

Housing and commercial property are still glutted with foreclosed and short sale inventory that keeps rolling into our market in Florida. Nevada and Ohio too. This too is improving.

In Florida foreclosures require a judge to rule for proceeding. That adds years to the banks full ownership process in abandoned houses. Although signs of nation wide recovery are showing up with a two percent gain in home values across the country overall with many resistant pockets.

New Bubbles with highs like twenty five percent gains in pricing are taking hold in some markets. So here we are five years past the 2008 Bush economic debacle, having solved a very real and looming worldwide bank collapse.

Banks were exposed as not having legitimate collateral, read insufficient income to service their debts. Congress voted to bail them out and most of the money has come back to the United States Treasury. The debacle of reselling the bundles of mortgages up and up the line, costing more and more, precipitated the housing collapse.

New homes are in demand in some markets. October 2012 closings on re-sales of existing homes are up twenty five percent from the month before.

In November 2012, the housing industry began a recovery with a two percent gain nationwide. President Obama is keeping us on course to recovery with no help from Congress. No programs get passed. There's no help for the housing industry like multiple Nationwide infrastructure projects to fix roads and bridges and create jobs.

Sadly the Republicans for Obama's first five years stood in opposition to all things Democratic placed for vote on the floor of the House of Representatives with a publicly stated priority to make President Obama a one term president, ha! Next best? Continue to be a do nothing Congress to make him a do nothing President his second term.

Like a discus thrower Obama launched and got passed in 2009 a somewhat truncated yet much better than nothing Affordable Health Care Act that is catching on with the American people. It's mandatory insurance starts January 2,2014. Small business start date, January 2, 2015.

ObamaCare depended on the election outcome being a Democratic win. Some House Republicans are still trying to repeal the Affordable Health Care Act, aka ObamaCare, having put the repeal to a vote in the House of Representatives in one form or another thirty three times and counting! Over forty four times and counting almost March, 2014.

The government is held hostage currently by the Tea Party Republicans. An imminent loss of funding of our national government spending money is threatened quite seriously by that segment of the GOP.

The House's GOP says funding the government is dependent on ObamaCare being unfunded!! How do the House of Representatives legislators see fit to capitulate to the hard liner Tea Partiers? The threat of well funded competition for their congressional seat back home. The Tea Party is funded by very deep pocketed individuals. Among others a pair of male siblings whose last name is Koch.

In 2012 we wondered if the hotly fought election would conclude cleanly remembering how ridiculously the United States Supreme Court got the job of naming the presidential winner in George W. Bush vs. Al Gore, 2000. That's another story.

Obama won his second term with fifty four percent of the popular vote and a significant margin of Electoral College Votes, those votes assigned state by state won variously.

The March 1, 2013 Sequestration across the board Federal cuts, came to be.

A pall hung over industry and worker alike, lunch programs and handicap transportation, too, for sometime before the realization of the lost funding. Results are proving highly problematic. More loss of compassion for the least among us is in the works. Republicans are on a march to squash health, meaning enough food to eat, and education out of the poorest peoples' reach. They want Food Stamp benefits cut by twenty percent and basic good Public Education possibly made unaffordable again.

Whisper: Are we being encouraged, raised, to become cheap labor and service personnel?

Under thirty two hour part time employees are everywhere. Impact is felt in every household affected.

Spending begets spending, not spending begets not spending. The part time employee spike is a show of rejection of the Affordable Care Act by capitalist corporations and entrepreneurs big and small who are reluctant to provide money for their employees health care.

It might not take long from a practical stance to see the cost benefits of employing people who see doctors and dentists in a timely fashion. Health care for those without is a big step up for our culture.

Doctors of Nutrition please step up with your guidance.

We are still struggling with getting the hungry fed even more than usual with recent program cuts meaning loss of funding.

We are dependent on a do nothing Congress to perform. Nothing was done from November 7th, 2012, the day after the election, through December 31, 2012.

President Obama won a second term, as you know. November 25th, 2012, a Monday, started the four weeks we watched carefully our Congress. In place was a long list of December 31st expirations to re-up or let drop. For example, reduced student loan interest rates, unemployment benefits period extensions, and primary home mortgage discrepancy money in short sale purchase considered as Taxable income, not forgiven as income without a Congressional ruling means an instant tax debt to the IRS for shortsale selling former homeowner. Without borrowed mortgage dollars left unpaid allowed income forgiveness, as unearned income necessarily waived, no longer IRS taxable income, the former homeowner selling unable to pay off the mortgage entirely, a shortsale, is stuck for multi thousands of surprise IRS debt.

Congress is behind approving the IRS shortsale income debt relief since the end of 2013 again this year 2014, Spring. They do these things any 'ol time and make them retroactive or not. Meanwhile how does one decide one's decisions for the future? If the game plan of our unable to function

Congress is to keep American citizenry off balance and Unnecessarily Uncertain, bulls eye.

Many government programs, like Meals on Wheels and Head Start, have Federal funding.

The eight percent sequestration cut currently does leave fifty seven thousand American children without the food aid that increases dramatically their calorie intake. The consequence of that calorie loss is a jeopardized future. That's what this money represents.

This unnecessary childhood hunger is our congressional representatives' fault. Not agreeing on the budget cuts caused their own crafted punishment to fall on many American heads, not theirs.

Months in, it's late September 2013. Kick in date for the sequestration was March 1, 2013, the on going consequence of the Sequestration to many is a lost job, wages.

It's important to see the connection between the handful of men in the 1930s who served as federal congressional legislators who were bamboozled by the nefarious, to do harm, in particular, the Marihuana Tax Act of 1937. We have again elected the bamboozled. The similarity is the repercussing harm done the American Public.

∧∧∧∧∧∧∧∧∧∧∧∧∧∧∧∧∧∧∧∧∧∧∧∧∧∧∧∧∧∧∧∧∧∧∧∧

Ahead of the general election in 2012, we voters could chose to revert to trickle down economics and deregulation again, that which lead America's and the world's financial health to a fiasco in 2008. At the time we really wondered if our teetering economy might topple the world's stability.

We want to find our way to firmer ground, not drastically cutting the budget in the immediate, imagining some over riding perk from a tiny bit more balanced budget would enhance us in the foreseeable future. Doing what hurts the many in the immediate, cutting funding and programs, reverts us back to seeing our hold on a financially solid ground future for the many disappear over the horizon.

The phoned in filibuster the Republicans use to empower the minority has become a hurdle. No gun law in the wake of the elementary school massacre in Connecticut, 2012.

No legislated background check at the point of sale of an automatic weapon, nothing passes. The debt ceiling issue is pushed to September 2013 and that's considered a major across the aisle victory to agree to pay our debts for a few months instead of weeks. The Republicans in Congress have been doing time consuming fights over doling small time increments of debt ceiling raising in order to insure anything productive could be ignored. Balderdash.

Thumbnail sketch of September 29, 2013, eve of the last day for The United States Congress to legislate backing off the United States Government's now partial, troops paid, Shut Down! Democrats are hanging tough to keep from the bad bargain offer of a year's delay on funding The Affordable Health Care Act also known as Obama Care. This from the Republicans' bossy Tea Party hardliners whose refusal to accept raising the debt ceiling is their give up if they can take away Obama Care. In the vernacular of old, "That's a hell of a note!"

osososososososososososososososo

Late September 2013 finds we the people battening down our whole government in anticipation of a Federal government Shut Down, plus possible defaults paying our bills. The threat to de-fund government effective October first knowing our low reserve ready cash lasts to mid October, meaning defaulting on incurred spending payments, has appeal to the Republican led House of Representatives. Our future collectively is being held hostage so the Democrats might cave and accept de-funding of The Affordable Health Care Act which launches October first, no matter what.

It costs billions of dollars, our dollars, to come through a Federal level government Shut Down. It was likely a milder shutdown impact when the mid nineteen nineties federal government shutdown took place.

It happened. October 1, 2013 the Feds shuttered up metaphysically for seventeen days and threw many bureaucratic functions into hiatus. The dire repercussions are with us still. Holiday sales paled. Home sales faltered. Federal employees and their work places languished. Major Tourist Attractions like our National Parks and Monuments, repelled visitors.

Reserve money existed back in the nineties to keep paying the bills longer for their government shutdown. Will this be our country's first actual debt default? Credibility debacle 'pile on' to ensue? Seventeen days into shutdown comes the debt ceiling raising necessity.

The deadline for raising the debt ceiling was met, barely. The shutdown ended as well. Seventeen days for the Republicans to feel the pain of gross unpopularity sufficiently to perform at last.

In January 2014 there's Major Hoopla over agreeing to accept a budget and debt ceiling raise to 2015. The House and Senate passed a bipartisan budget for the first time since 2008. The president signed it, December, 2013.

ososososososososososososososososososo

Late October 2012, Super Storm, Hurricane Sandy, an eight hundred mile wide huge cyclonic event, hit the northeast United States a devastating wallop. New Jersey went without power for so many for weeks. Restoration of the state is bound to take months to years. Lower Manhattan, Staten Island, the least above sea level for all the northeast got a flood impact. Our Federal government is stepping up mightily to aid in a quick recovery where possible. Damage may top a trillion dollars at the end, or close.

It took two votes to pry the money out of the Republican Congress for the aid New Jersey needed after Hurricane Sandy, November 2012.

Much of the boardwalk was open for business on the Jersey Shore in time for the Memorial Day holiday weekend, 2013.

Hurricane Sandy turned conversation to climate change, yes or no. Science supports yes, saying fossil fuel exhaust and our prodigious pollution is fueling climate change. Ninety five percent of scientists weighing in agree. Ninety five percent of the pollution is humon attributed. Verify these two facts.

Climate change explained: Our pollution has heat to cause icebergs in the Artic Circle to melt. More and colder water moves farther south than ever. Simply, weather is the interaction of warming and cooling currents of air and warming and cooling currents of water. We experience more cooling and more extreme weather events farther south because of the colder water in our oceans.

Antarctica is growing wetter too.

wearezoomininonourwin

The passion and money are with the status quo, however. The top moneyed industry whose top dog, Exxon Mobile, likes a fossil fuel based economy.

We had heard in the election rhetoric that a new Republican administration would be giving the Federal Emergency Management Authority, FEMA, it's walking papers in favor of a subsidy to each state to do the job. That's not looking practical in the light of the recent eight hundred mile wide storm event, Hurricane Sandy, impacting many states in the north eastern sector.

Shrinking government participation in our lives is an untimely proposition at this juncture for so many reasons.

We are the people. While we are left to observe the diminishing governmental support for those needing it most we may feel helpless. Administrations have the soft belly of public scrutiny. The public has the ability to speak out for equal rights and justice.

Yes, the November 2012 election dust settled with Obama winning. The House of Representatives still a Republican slightly slimmer majority with a continued Democratic Senate majority, by a narrow margin. We, indeed, have to keep gritting our teeth as we watch the Republicans block compromise to any legislation that if passed would work for we the people's well being.

Congress doing nothing is interpreted as a legitimate successful strategy nowadays, go figure. It's the best they can do for the country. Huh?

At the very least, any Supreme Court Justices appointed by Obama will not likely be in the mold of Justice Scallia, the far right conservative judge, as Obama's opponent in his bid for a second term, the ex-Massachusetts Governor Mitt Romney, promised.

Our Supreme Court is so huge in determining our quality of life this Democratic second term is a major victory. Momentum may be building for another Democratic win in 2016 and ought to be so, based on this Supreme Court new Judge appointee issue alone.

Anonymous contributors as the biggest donors to electoral campaigns are new this election, thanks to a Supreme Court ruling.

Looking ahead, diplomacy at the helm, with luck there won't be a war to fight. If there is, it will be the depleted middle class that will pay with blood and treasure, again. Syria is problematical. It's dictator did use chemical weapons against his people seeking his ouster, apparently. Diplomacy took a leap of faith and created space for a solution to the dictator's savagery. Calm came quickly out of the diplomacy of the magnifying glass. Secretary of State John Kerry stays the course.

Syria is dissolving into many factions working individually to unseat an implacable sitting dictator running the military. Migration out of Syria is in the millions. Temporary camps are becoming permanent as the flow of humonity exiting Syria builds. Each hosting country despairs.

The Ukraine has erupted. Here is a country torn by ethnic divides and political loyalties. The Russian half versus the western/European leaning half. One has the Russian language the other English. Bad Dictator left the country for Russia.

Their former Dictator's extravagance has broken the Ukraine people's economy. Russian troops come in and the free world demands they leave. Fresh Crisis, March 7, 2014.

The Crimea has been annexed by Russia without much ado.

Occupation, quick dubiously legal referendum vote and done.

Still March 2014.

*6*7*8*6*7*8*6*7*8*6*7*8*6*

The bottom line for conservatives subconsciously or not is a cheap labor force for the 'job creators'. Their solutions could have this 'unintended' consequence equaling goodbye middle class. Defunding libraries and schools is no way to compete on a global scale.

When the first satellite in space was Russia's Sputnik, nicely successfully launched, our leadership went into overdrive to have all manner of Americans get more education. We had to grow the expertise in science and technology to compete. We did and launched the first man in space and put a man on the moon in less than a decade.

The growing gap between the haves and have nots educationally is our current dilemma. Due to our self imposed budget restraints we find ourselves dropping in the ranks among nations, our students lacking the skills and knowledge other countries' children have. We are not even close to the top ten in anything evaluated.

If the ultra conservatives have their way it will take about three generations for American children to grow up struggling not to be those migrating from harvest to harvest for a lifetime, unless they like that life.

Could be mechanical harvesting will be fully implemented by then.

More liberal forces seek making pre-school to higher education affordable and accessible to make climbing the ladder of economic success open to the many. Liberals believe health care in a wealthy nation belongs as a birthright. Nutrition and basic care for all of us strengthens us all. That's a better outcome than leaving to chance a distressed population crippled by health care cost burdens and losing production ability over inadequate food fueling whether a baby, reduced for life, or a hungry senior scaling up eventual health care costs.

In this battle for territory, the rich secure their wealth by not sharing in general and blindly accepting the existing blueprint for wealth acquisition, fossil fuel, doctored cows, Cannabis as a Schedule 1 Classified Drug.

The status quo. Shareholders enjoy their oblivion.

Privilege has it's privileges and the poor we will always have with us. Well, not necessarily. We can fix inequities in our tax code. Separate Church and State. Collect tax on the land religion owns. Doesn't have to be huge money at first. Stop subsidizing the oil industry. Scrape the advantages making big businesses tax free.

We can make the least among us educated and ready for the best opportunity they can uncover. We can move on to true cradle to grave health care beginning with a single birth from a specific not too distant date. We may get to the point where we provide the opportunity for a classy education to all willing and able to do the work.

Suppose we focus on imagination and growth and decide to allow individuals to live without borders with simple rules for boundaries in place mainly for tax paying purposes.

America is great because it has a life force of it's own that thrives on Freedom and Truth. We don't want to sink farther from prosperity. We have the ability to track our way to good health, good educations and good opportunity without favoring the rich. Choose knowledge over hyper emotion to use as guide.

As it happens the first legislated persecution of drug users began legislatively as the Harrison Act of 1914. It passed ignoring the case made against the legislation by doctors and The American Medical Association itself.

The Harrison Act also known as the Narcotics Act of 1914 turned hard drugs, opiates from poppies and cocaine from the coca plant, into contraband on the spot. History teaches us the motive behind the law had to do with China's opiate problems, our discrimination against the Chinese in America and our opiate issues in our newly acquired Philippines. The Chinese put a trade embargo in place against America. The Narcotics criminalizing Harrison Act of 1914 evolved from 1906 to 1911 to 1913 to Woodrow Wilson's inauguration and signing the Act into law February 8,1914.

The Act imposed record keeping for cocaine and opiate transactions. The Treasury Department enforced the law by pursuing druggists and physicians who maintained opiate and cocaine addicted patients. Doctors were penalized if they provided the treatment of weaning addicts off their drug. Deaths from opiate and cocaine use and the number of users both tripled in as many months.

Rumors said Negros in the South required bigger bullets to be shot dead once they did cocaine. The idea that drugs enhance a person's prowess proved intimidating. Afro American Pot users were also said to be better marksmen with Pot than peers without Pot.

August 24th, 2013 Washington DC hosted a commemoration of Martin Luther King's "I have a Dream." speech right there where he delivered the speech fifty years prior. Many many thousands of respectful individuals graced the mall. The speeches made mention of the trials of the current day.

Voting rights depravations are no longer over as seen in typically divisive states like Texas. The Supreme Court has reversed portions of the Voter's Rights Law. It's an uphill climb now to stay as good as it just was. The Federal Justice Department in reaction to this early 2014 ruling is determined to go all out protecting voting rights state by state, per Attorney General Eric Holder.

.,.,.,.,.,.,.,.,.

Before the Harrison Act was passed by Congress, on December 14th, 1914, The New York Times published an article entitled "Negro Cocaine 'fiends' Are New Southern Menace: Murder and Insanity Increasing Among Lower-Class Blacks" by Edward Huntington Williams which reported that Southern sheriffs had increased the caliber of their weapons from .32 to .38 to bring down Negros under the effect of cocaine. [See Thomas, Evan (September 15,1986). America's Crusade"; Time Magazine.]

Now look at every negative popular belief demonizing Pot such as 'it makes a person brain dead'. In truth, we all have our built in receptors for THC in our brains and the results of feeding our brain's receptors THC are uniformly positive, to devotees.

Take each so called reason ever stated said to explain why Pot Heads are inferior, nay, criminal people, and turn it around. The best lie is the one directly contrary to the truth. Consider the media support like a drumbeat's repeat over decades stating a lie to make us believers. Ask why.

Corporate ownership of the media and sponsors like Pfizer Pharmaceutical back United States Congressmun. Many moneyed interests lobby to protect the interests of big business from competition from a beneficial Weed that is actually a multi fold asset to the humon condition.

The facts are out there. Google Tetrahydrocannabinol, also known as THC, for the science behind Pot, Cannabis, Marihuana. Discover the attributes of Pot's psychoactive ingredient, THC.

When the receptors in our brains for THC, get THC, our brains store and treasure it. We may test positive for Cannabis for months after the last consumption. Alcohol and cocaine are treated like the poison they are by the body. They are expelled from the body as quickly as possible. At the highest degree of saturation of alcohol in the body, short of death, how long to dump it entirely? About two to three days. Alcohol, cocaine, nicotine and caffeine are all four common physically addictive drugs meaning a very hard habit to break because the body sickens without the drug.

The, oh, so popular, DRUG CAFFEINE in coffee and Coke and Pepsi and all the rest, more softly in Chocolate, causes the brain to grow caffeine receptors. The down sides of alcohol, nicotine and cocaine are not news. Caffeine teamed with alcohol is a current trend. This legal libation combo claims our young as victims quickly. Such deaths have made the newspaper headlines. Death by alcohol combined with caffeine became a news alert January 2012.

For Comparison purposes: Alcohol is a physical depressant that can kill an over zealous drinker in less than twenty four hours. Laced with caffeine, even quicker, because more alcohol, in less time, is consumed. Should the inebriated attempt to drive a car it means innocent people may become victims of another's alcohol impairment. About ten thousand innocent Americans die annually due to drunk drivers. An untallied additional thousands and thousands are damaged. The ten thousand deaths number is a big improvement. Deaths by driving drunks went down almost twenty percent from the high due to the outrage and measures taken. Only now there has been no change in the ten thousand dead annually at the hands of merciless drunks, for fifteen years, 2013.

Alcohol consumption past a bare minimum, a few ounces a day only, is a risk factor for every disease except maybe the illness caused by eating contaminated raw oysters. The alcohol may kill the bacteria in the stomach, before it takes residence in the gut in the instance of eating bad oysters. And alcohol could be helpful if something happens and you are totally passed out and this keeps you oblivious and incapacitated at a time when awake and alert won't do.

Alcohol is the root cause of so much violence, especially domestically.

Alcohol is said to cause over half of all Domestic Violence. It's said the police called to stem such say it's the most terrifying part of their work at least up until it's determined no one else is armed at the scene of the domestic violence. More than fifty percent of all domestic violence is attributed to alcohol consumption.

Yet we are able to tolerate and socialize easily with alcohol and somewhat still, tobacco. We allow ourselves to forget how alcohol damages the unborn forever, kills our livers, and ruins innocent lives and careers and marriages routinely, directly and peripherally. Alcohol use should be well ahead of Pot use if you want to be angry at your youngsters for a forbidden 'pleasure'.

It's wiser to be truthful if you want to be believed.

Beer, any alcoholic beverage, may be every adolescent boy and girl's rite of passage in our culture. Why, you may wonder, is tolerance of a kinder gentler option, that's not physically addictive, denied? For what reason?

>9797979797979797979797979797<

Note: Cocaine and all the other drugs classified as contraband, plus prostitution and gambling as consumed, are part of the humon condition. We are all best served to _not_ exclude the people who want them or provide them. Once we grow into loving and caring people as a whole we will abandon Contraband Gangsterism, Contraband Markets. Those choices make matters worse only.

Generally accepted as Legally created, Contraband Markets for narcotics and contraband desired services create systemic bribes, kickbacks and even more General Corruption by virtue of bestowing HIDDEN UNTAXED SUPER WEALTH on Outlaws, Criminals, and Thugs who simply keep adding untapped consumers by staying current with trends if not manipulating the latest drug trends into being.

Is it humone to turn over an entire segment of our population to be caught as outlaws within the contraband industry and it's opposition? So many Americans are left with no recourse to police help if they are crime victims themselves.

We the people skirt the obvious. The United States Congress is not empowered to make criminals out of Cannabis Aficionados. Making Cannabis contraband and illegal is another erroneous and bad, likely unconstitutional, policy Law. Separating an individual in public from contraband may be enforceable as a successful Congressional law for now. But booking anyone with Cannabis, separating them from their

Liberty, is an indefensible humon rights violation. Congress may not criminalize a subset of American citizenry without cause legally. Criminality of otherwise innocent individuals to be legal criminality must be passed as such by two thirds of our State Legislators per state. Passed as an Amendment to our United States Constitution. Because this has not been done we remain bamboozled by an historical wrong. All of us suffer the consequences of the implementation of an implied only, non existent law, requiring an Amendment to our United States Constitution to be legitimate.

Our legal institutions stand revealed as nefarious by willfully not serving the public in this matter, but instead enjoying the business.

This is easily remedied with the facts of Congressional limitations finally commonly known.

Wemun as 'drug' convicted prisoners serve longer sentences than the men they were caught with in general.

The men in the bust have names to give up for reduced sentencing. The more associates named the fewer years to serve.

From tainted contraband goods (not Pot) bought and imbibed by a Princeton Freshman to the battered and left for dead sex worker in Queens; why not help the freshmun up front with vendor accountability, legal purchase and sale. Let the Sex Worker make a call to 911 for help anywhere anytime. The Sex Worker working monitored for accountability by virtue of the sex service being a legal purchase and sale. Picture calm out of chaos.

!#!#!#!#!#!#!#!#!#!#!#!

Portugal has for all practical purposes allowed consumption of the usual contraband drugs for the last decade plus. Doing so solved the ramped up excessive public use evident in Portugal in 2002. In 2012, we learn the Portuguese are pleased with the reversal of the problem legalizing brought, by and large. Worth further study.

Tobacco. It's all been said. Don't. If you already do, quit. The day is coming when all smoking will take place in private. Not even on the open road will tobacco or any smoking be allowed. No more riding down the road, car window down, hanging a burning cigarette out the window.

Self driving cars to the rescue.

In California people do have legal access to Cannabis venders and growers. There, vendors are selling, besides the usual resiney buds, edibles and topicals laced with Cannabis. It's supposed to replace smoking it entirely. Thank you California.

Denver, Colorado has recently granted well over three hundred vendor or grower licenses ahead of the legal January 1, 2014 recreational Pot usage voted into existence in 2012. Wow.

)#)#)#)#)#)#)#(#(#(#(#(#(#(

Busting the Gateway Drug Myth:

The individual in the Gateway Drug Myth discovers that the Herb turned illicit 'Drug' does not transform doobie smokers into fiends, addicts, criminals, thieves, or even academic misfits, or under performers.

So why not try Cocaine? Why should that be different? In the myth scenario the pusher is going to move the person into a hard drug habit because they can. Here's the catch, the myth depends on the purchase source to be professionally selling hard drugs. Marihuana is not commonly bought on the street or asking the wrong stranger.

Most first encounters to Cannabis is Cannabis shared with them by a trusted friend. The supply chain is as grass roots as grass roots implies. The Popularity of Cannabis, also once called Grass, depends on performance, not professional Public Relations campaigns.

This supply chain of local people is not likely to have a pipeline to opiates and pharmaceuticals. Be an alcoholic or almost alcoholic enjoying the legal walk in service of a Bar Life and you could find yourself seduced by a real drug pusher, so don't do that.

In some markets, okay New York City, Cannabis delivery to one's door is available, or has been. Kind of like Domino's Pizza. Keep in mind nowhere is Marihuana Policy/Law not present. There is a 'law tripwire of culpability', where ever you are, equally unjustly, early December, 2013.

The South American country Uruguay is stepping up as the first whole country exception providing a legalization policy for all residents as of mid December, 2013. Another Wow.

Oregon and Colorado legalized Cannabis in the voting booth November, 2012.

Provided the Federal Prosecutors in the states with legal Cannabis follow the recently established Federal Guideline to not prosecute a Federal law that jeopardizes the legal legislation in their respective state relating to Cannabis, Federal prosecution over Cannabis is finished in those states. Big WOW.

In that event, you know which you are perhaps. You are now, or by January 1, 2014, able to relax. Your non criminal status at acquisition is whole and complete. At present it is policy for all of us to have the protection of privacy as defined by the 'American homes are our personal castles' pervasive constitutional take.

On a related topic, the NSA, the National Security Agency eavesdroppers extraordinaire, stand revealed. Of course the United States Supreme Court has ruled concerning the NSA's work of constant surveillance of all our electronic communication as constitutional. It became a Supreme Court case in 2013.

Some judges say the search for terrorists is a good enough excuse. Another agrees the people have privacy guarantees for the NSA to honor. At present there is an unregulated legal limitation of the NSA to a terrorist hunt which appears blown through by an NSA revealed search selective of people into internet porn. Ug. Metadata it's called. All of everything goes into the NSA net. Detailed results of any kind are available.

efukkuffukkuffukkuffuke

Firefighters like Cannabis for stress relief and lung health. Adult lives call for de-stressing. Being something that is so called 'psychologically addictive' translates to mean that at whatever point an individual who regularly gets high on Cannabis, or stoned, should that individual determine to stop, has run out, is too busy, wants to pass a pee test, or did get busted, whatever the circumstance, that individual, suffers no withdrawal symptoms from day one. Lament, could be.

Exceptions do exist and seeking professional help is worthwhile for those exceptions. A general satisfaction concerning Cannabis exists for most Cannabis people with or without the Herb. With is just better, healthier to some. Maybe most all.

Coffee, Cola, any caffeine regular use, even chocolate? Yes, even chocolate, stop cold and possibly experience headache, lethargy and relapses galore. Nicotine withdrawals are now managed by laboratory products to ooze drugs into you through a commercially sold patch placed on the skin like a square band aide. No end of services are offered. The folks who are afflicted with a physical addiction have their own interventions, recovery devices, institutions etc. Many treatments are covered by insurance so we all pay.

March 2014, first responders carry a device that sprays into a victim's mouth the anecdote to a deadly heroin overdose. The individual then revives back to life. It seems that the recent stepped up policing to stop pharmaceutical painkiller pill trafficking has caused the recent heroin escalation in heroin users and many deaths. Family members can buy Narcam to have handy to save a known heroin addicted relative. The price was under twenty five dollars per unit and is now about double due to demand.

Cannabis? No toxins. An asset to the humon condition. No Patents. Competes well. Sold illegally. Until soon.

January 1,2014 in Colorado the taxing of Cannabis sales begins. Full legality. The Feds are not going to intervene with prosecutions unless some Federal prosecuter rebels. 2013, it's still a wait and see.

alalalalalalalalalalalalala

THE GATEWAY DRUGS:

I.   Inhaled TOBACCO, LOWERS RESISTANCE TO
     INHALING anything.

Tobacco also places an individual on the shunned vulnerable side more and more, especially for the underprivileged hanging out.

In the case of Pot one never knows what it is one inhales as there are no consumer protections in place unless one personally knows the grower or has a connoisseur's nose. Fortunately, Pot is abundant and not tempting to tamper with on a large scale, nor does it spoil easily. Knowing the truth about Pot removes the fear of ill conceived wrong doing.

II. BOOZE, All Alcohol, Lowers, to WIPES OUT, the
     drinker's INHIBITIONS by diminishing the alcohol
     consumer's functional abilities, cognitive and physical.
     Poor Judgment ensues. Alcoholics in the last stages
     of alcohol deterioration suffer Delirium Tremens'
     or serious hallucinations, thus the proverbial Pink
     Elephants commonly mentioned as descriptive of what
     an advanced alcoholic describes seeing.

Back to the individual who likely tries Pot by sharing a pipe bowl full or a paper rolled joint with a trusted friend. Should that person want to acquire their own supply, what to do? Go to the same source as the friend. Or mention you tried it and like the occasional Pot High to someone you know. Through them you find a connection.

Head Shops sold paraphernalia back in the seventies and have staged a comeback of sorts. One may peruse the local tobacco store for rolling papers and pipes. Popular now is the Hookah, similar to the many limbed water pipe of the giant mushroom sitting caterpillar of Alice in Wonderland fame.

A Hookah is sold for use with the fragrance treated tobacco enjoyed in private clubs and by home party enthusiasts. This swiftly creates many fresh nicotine addicts practically on the spot. It would be nice to have apparatus legally sold meant for inhaling cooled Cannabis.

Keep in mind that it is feloniously illegal paraphernalia once you partner Cannabis with your Hookah.

We are kept from getting relief in the courts. Suppose the defendant opts for or is required to have a traditional trial. Prospective jurors are 'legitimately' culled through as to their will to convict based on the possession facts presented matching the law for a conviction. Where as juries historically had the intrinsic power in the courtroom once the judge gave them the case for deliberation. They could nullify. A jury was able to set precedent, able to set free anyone who was deemed to be a Not Guilty by virtue of not meeting the standard of what truly constitutes criminal behavior by definition and practice, common sense.

Our legislators have provided rules forcing judges to imprison the convicted according to Draconian sentencing guidelines. Irrevocable sentencing guidelines. The contracts to build prisons went flying out the door until the national security business took off after 9/11 and Drug courts came along. Drug Courts began in Miami, Dade County, in the eighties. Further Drug Court details as you read.

Tuesday, March 15, 2011, C-Span aired our newest Federal Head of the Corrections Department at the podium. He was introduced with the words he was bringing "exciting" news of policy shifts. It turns out he is aware of the people out of prison with their rights never reinstated for life because they are convicted felons.

"There are Felons, and there are Felons," The Attorney General said.

He wanted the audience to know that some felons are not bad and if we differentiate, the good ones will get back the right to vote and perhaps to no longer be discriminated against routinely and eliminated from employment at the application threshold as they are now. They never get to the pee test.

Does Obama's Attorney General Eric Holder mean to say there are felons who deserve to be convicted and those that never should have been arrested in the first place? Their offence being in actuality, politically motivated as a long standing unlawful discrimination against possession of a medicinal Creation Given Natural Resource that functions as a Health Restorative, a scientifically factual description. Ask doctors in the Medical Marihuana twenty states plus the District of Columbia, better known as Washington DC. Ask the doctors in the states that already allow Medical Marijuana. Understand, Pot arrests and the fear of same, ending in incarceration or not, are all Persecution.

Listed here are the twenty United States of America plus Washington DC, the District of Columbia, with State Legal only, Federally Illegal less but still, Medical Marijuana.

Colorado and Washington State, have recreational use okay too, up to one ounce per individual. Freedom as passed November Elections, 2012. Implementation pending tax collection roll out effective January 2014. News, May 19, 2013.

1. Alaska, 1998, Ballot Measure 8(58%)$25/$20 fees, limit 1 usable ounce, 6 plants;

2. <u>Arizona</u>, 2010 Proposition 203(50.13%)$150/75 fees, 2.5 usable ounces, 0-12 plants;

3. <u>California,</u> 1996, Proposition 215 (56%) $66/$33, 8 usable ounces, 6 mature plants;

4. <u>Colorado</u>, 2000, Ballot Amendment 20 (54%) $35, 2 usable ounces, 6 plants;

5. <u>Connecticut</u>, 2012 House Bill 5389 (96-51 House, 21-13 Senate) no fee, One-month supply (as determined);

6. <u>DC</u>, 2010, Amendment Act B18-622 (13-0 vote) no fees, 2 dried ounces, limits on???;

7. <u>Delaware</u>, 2011, Senate Bill 17 (27-14 House, 17-4 Senate) no fees, 6 usable ounces;

8. <u>Hawaii</u>, 2000, Senate Bill 862 (32-18 House, 13-12 Senate) $25, 3 usable ounces, 7 plants;

9. <u>Illinois,</u> 2013, House Bill 1 (61-57 House; 35-21 Senate)Fee TBD, 2.5 oz. usable; 6 plants;

10. <u>Maine</u>, 1999 Ballot Question 2 (61%) $100/$75, 2.5 usable Ounces, 6 plants;

11. <u>Massachusetts</u>, 2012, Ballot Question 2 (63%) Fee TBD, Sixty day supply for personal use;

12. <u>Michigan</u>, 2008, Proposal 1 (63%) $100/$25,2.5 usable ounces, 12 plants;

13. <u>Montana</u>, 2004, Initiative 148 (62%) $25/$10, 1 usable ounce, 4 plants;

14. <u>Nevada</u>, 2000 Ballot Question 9 (66%) $200+ fees, 1 usable ounce, 7 plants;

15. <u>New Hampshire</u>, 2013, House Bill 573 (284-66 House, 18-6 Senate) Fee TBD, two ounces of useable Cannabis during a 10 day period;

16. <u>New Jersey</u>, 2010, Senate Bill 119 (48-14 House, 25-13 Senate)$200+ fees, 2 usable ounces;

17. <u>New Mexico</u>, 2007 Senate Bill 523 (36-31 house, 32-3 Senate) $0, 6 usable ounces, 16 plants;

18. <u>Oregon</u>, 1998, Ballot Measure 57 (55%) $200/$100,24 usable ounces, 9 plants;

19. <u>Rhode Island</u>, 2006, Senate Bill 0710 (52-10 House, 33-1 Senate) $75/$10, 2.5 usable ounces, 12 plants;

20. <u>Vermont</u>, 2004 Senate Bill 76 (22-7)HB 645 (82-59), 2 usable ounces, 9 plants;

21. <u>Washington</u>, 1998 Initiative 692 (59%) no fee, 24 usable ounces, 15 plants.

22. Maryland, 2014 May, State Governor moves to allow Medical Marihuana.

<u>Hallucinate</u>; experience a seemingly real perception of something not actually present, typically as a result of a mental disorder or of taking drugs. <u>Hallucination</u>; An experience involving the perception of something not present. Hallucinatory; of or resembling a hallucination; inducing hallucinations. <u>Hallucinogen</u>; a drug such as LSD that causes Hallucinations. Definitions as found in <u>The Oxford American College Dictionary</u>, published in 2002.

Weed does not cause hallucinations. Seeing or hearing what is not there is not part of the Weed High. The entertainment value of what one sees on the back of one's eyelids when one closes one's eyes may be enhanced.

Perhaps you've heard of the Rainbow Connection? Hearsay has it Jim Henson of Muppet Fame could explain. When one's Cannabinal quotient is at saturation say, it's easy to see a color or two or three from the rainbow on a pale reflecting lighted surface. The color patterns if not all glistening or moving are a kind of reflection shaping to the surface observed. Tiles might pattern out pink and yellow. It has to do with the light and the ability to see what's there to be seen, just like the rainbow, seeable sometimes under the right conditions. There's a lot of natural light here now and the Computer screen has a pleasant fine stationary look of muted dabbles of pink and yellow all over for fleeting moments and gone or sustaining.

Every color is every where, there to be seen.

red.orange.yellow.green.blue.indigo.violet

It appears one of the main functions of the active ingredients in Cannabis is to facilitate oxygen to the brain for enhanced function. A brain with enhanced oxygen is a better brain. That's science. The usual mood elevation that characterizes a Cannabis high is the proof we are to indulge. THC is the active ingredient in Cannabis. We all have THC receptors. We are all born with them in our brains in many separate locations, the frontal lobe, thinking, the hypothalamus, emotions and the cortex, memory.

Ask any medical doctor what percent of their scripts are for mood elevation. Every single one of the patented prescribed laboratory made drugs, like Paxil, has negative side effects whether those negative side effects are pronounced enough to cause trouble or not. Without exception. The ads on TV, the print ads that want you to ask your doctor about their pill for your condition must state the potential very bad or not so bad consequences to your body that could ensue should you take the advertised prescription drug. The possible side effects sound devastating. Who would risk all those potential dire consequences, the worst being sudden death. Sometimes you have too wonder. . . ?

Could numerous industries feel threatened by a freely legal and home grow-able and mushrooming legal Pot vender industry?

To name a few of the perhaps threatened, Beer, Wine, All Alcohol, All tobacco, Health Care, Pharmaceuticals, Pee testers, Law Enforcement, gear for Law enforcement, Big Cancer, Drug courts! Including the GIGANTIC Bureaucracy receiving the Drug War dole.

Remember too, property belonging to a convicted Pot grower or purveyor likely will be confiscated by law enforcement and may be sold to enrich law enforcement coffers. This serves to strip any accumulated asset wealth from a felonious act. In every other felony conviction do thieves have to lose their houses? Bought with ill gotten gains or not?

Here is a list of what our United States Congress has over time accomplished on behalf of winning the Drug War, so to speak.

1. "Controlled Substances Act" October, 27,1970.
   This one is the foundation of all else here. All the following are in reverse order, first the most recent then chronologically going back to 1970.
2. "Secure and Responsible Drug Disposal Act of 2010"
3. "Combat Methamphetamine Enhancement Act of 2010"
4. "Fair Sentencing Act of 2010"
5. "Methamphetamine Production Prevention Act of 2008"
6. "Combat Methamphetamine Epidemic Act of 2005"
7. "Controlled Substances Export Reform Act of 2005"
8. "Anabolic Steroid Control Act of 2004"

Insert: Each of these thirty six may well have funding for a study and/or a committee with a uniform two years to sunset and report, unless extended. These funds are allocated to various and sundry existing Bureaucratic Institutions like the Secretary of State to Congressional committees to newly formed auspices, perhaps within service, civil or federal, for example, the Coast Guard. Lots of programs, lots of flowing tax payer dollars.

9. "Illicit Drug Anti-Proliferation Act of 2003"
10. "Drug Addiction Treatment Act of 2000"
11. "Methamphetamine Anti-Proliferation Act of 2000"
12. "Hillary J. Fairies and Samantha Reid Date-Rape Drug Prohibition Act"
13. "Western Hemisphere Drug Elimination Act"
14. "Controlled Substances Trafficking Prohibition Act" November 10,1998.
15. "Drug-Induced Rape Prevention and Punishment Act of 1996"
16. "Comprehensive Methamphetamine Control Act of 1996"
17. "Drug Free Truck Stop Act", September 13,1994.
18. "Domestic Chemical Diversion Control Act of 1993"
19. "Anabolic Steroids Control Act of 1990"
20. "Anti-Drug Abuse Amendments Act of 1988"
21. "Chemical Diversion and Trafficking Act of 1988"
22. "Asset Forfeiture Amendments Act of 1988"
23. "Anti-Drug Abuse Act of 1986"
24. "Narcotics Penalties and Enforcement Act of 1986"
25. "Drug Possession Penalty Act of 1986"
26. "Juvenile Drug Trafficking Act of 1986"
27. "Controlled Substance Analogue Enforcement Act of 1986"
28. "Continuing Drug Enterprises Act of 1986"

29. "Controlled Substances Import and Export Penalties Enhancement Act of 1986"
    By 1986's conclusion; seven Acts!
30. "Mail Order Drug Paraphernalia Control Act", November 29, 1990 AS REPEALED... begun between '84 & '86
31. "Controlled Substances Penalties Amendments Act of 1984"
32. "Dangerous Drug Diversion Control Act of 1984"
33. "Psychotropic Substances Act of 1978"
34. "Narcotic Addict Treatment Act of 1974"
35. "Comprehensive Drug Abuse Prevention and Control Act of 1970"
36. Repeat of #1 : also known as the "Controlled Substances Act", October 27, 1970.
    Short title: "Controlled Substances Import and Export Act" which enacted subchapter II of this Chapter of the law.

See below, as dated, shown as located on page 10 of 270, as printed, as found, of what pulls up searching United States Congressional "Drug Abuse Prevention and Control Act of 1970", Here see the top of page one:

-CITE-
21 UNITED STATES CONGRESS CHAPTER 13 - DRUG ABUSE PREVENTION AND CONTROL 01/03/2012 (112-90)

-EXPCITE-
TITLE 21 - FOOD and DRUGS
CHAPTER 13 - DRUG ABUSE PREVENTION AND CONTROL

-Head-

CHAPTER 13 - DRUG ABUSE PREVENTION AND CONTROL

-MISCI-

SUBCHAPTER I - CONTROL AND ENFORCEMENT

Further delving will be from Subchapter II!

Seen below as printed: SEVERABILITY

Invalid or Unenforceable: "Any provision of this title {see Short title of 2000 Amendments note above} held to be invalid or unenforceable by its terms, or as applied to any person or circumstance, shall be construed as to give the maximum effect permitted by law, <u>unless such provision is held to be utterly invalid and unenforceable, in which event such provision shall be severed from this title</u> and shall not affect the applicability of the remainder of this title, or of such provision, to other persons not similarly situated or to other, dissimilar circumstances." The End.

We are all for the severance of Marijuana from the law.
Could this be the way out? Shall Marijuana be severed from this Title? {Title being the shorthand word for this 270 page document, as exerted from and shown above.}

Other non act programs as excerpted from and shown here from the 270 page Drug Abuse Prevention and Control-1970 Law:

1. Continuation of Orders, Rules and Regulations: a mere Statement.

2. Anti-Drug Messages on Federal Government Internet Sites as shall be controlled by the National Aeronautics and Space Administration, as consulting the Office of National Drug Control Policy. October 30, 2000.

3. Awareness Campaign: the Attorney General and Drug Enforcement Administration and the Federal Bureau of Investigation get to model protocols, pay grants at The Attorney General's discretion for forensic field Tests to detect the presence of gamma hydroxybutyric acid And related substances, appropriate funds allocated.

What is that? And I know I missed the awareness part of the campaign. Also included, 'designer drugs'.

opsopsopsopsopsopsopsopsops

Amazing that nature would provide a simple herb, Pot, with so many positive applications. Plus Pot grows like a weed. And Marihuana's only negative side effect stems exclusively from the misplaced perceived need to have it continue to be contraband. No hallucinations. One does see The Rainbow Connection quite literally occasionally. A surface will reveal a surface reflection showing yellow or yellow and violet on say, the computer screen, a tile floor. Your own skin in just the right light, will show the whole rainbow of color. It's what is there all the time. The light has to illuminate and the eye must look and the mind sees the reflection or however one sees rainbows themselves, moisture and light just right. Classification as an hallucinogen comes from an effect something may have in the brain that appears to stimulate one's optical capacity. A drunkard in the last stages of the DTs, Delirium Tremors, experiences hallucinations, hence the Pink Elephant illusion we often hear. LSD was said to be Hallucinogenic by those taking it. The mind would be so stimulated in such a way that the mind could not make practical sense of the flush of new perceptions yet attempts to make known the unknown. The problem was the breach between ill formed wrong perceptions and reality that results in or causes extreme LSD highs to upset takers due to overwhelming distorting misperceptions. Too far out. Individuals on LSD make drastic errors. They might think they can fly. That being the most publicized extreme reaction. Not a good lab drug for general consumption, most everyone agrees.

Conversely, Pot is a delicate miraculous blend of physical, mental and emotional asset just waiting to come to our aid.

Think of the time long long ago and maybe not so far far away when a forest might be burning and all the living creatures downwind from the moving on the wind fire would inhale the fragrant Cannabis burning with the forest or brush on a plain, and find therefore the necessary mental ability and physical endurance and will to save themselves.

A health restorative that grows like a weed and can't be patented poses an unparalleled legitimate competitive threat to Big Pharmaceutical Concerns that produce lab made health aids, pain killers, such as Advil and Tylenol. Thus the relentless demonizing. Marihuana is not a miracle cure for all users. No one anything will ever be that.

Tylenol users may not exceed the recommended dosage without risking being in immediate danger. A Study done by the FDA recently revealed the danger. A warning is about to go in place on the Packaging of Tylenol. One ingredient, acetaminophen, destroys humon liver function surprisingly quickly when consumed in moderate excess.

People of twenty states, in the face of an ongoing Federal contrabaning of Pot, still in place, saw fit to allow Marihuana, based on commonly held knowledge, to be made legally available by prescription. Two states are taking the plunge to Cannabis legalization, Colorado Hooray!

Hooray Washington! Voted on and passed November 2012.

Yes, a Wonderful Surprise! The 2012 November elections shone a bright light on reform. The people of Colorado and Washington state both passed legalization of RECREATIONAL MARIHUANA! The winds of change are upon us.

December 14, 2012, President Obama said publicly the Federal government will no longer bother with Pot smokers as "there are bigger fish to fry." Still the DEA strikes when and where it pleases to raid and arrest commercial Pot ventures.

Dawns a new day! The chink in the wall of exclusion is a widening space. The tossed handful of snow in a ball is balling up into an avalanche of acceptance of truth. The Feds say a tax mechanism for the purchase of the state legal one ounce per adult person is in the works for Colorado. People in Portland, Oregon had another smoke-in, August 2013. With this change to legal Cannabis one would no longer need a prescription to be served at a dispensary of Cannabis, although this year's first quarter marks a time when the prescription will save you fifty percent at the dispensary cash register, no plastic or checks, please.

First week of December 2013 Floridians are treated to much media coverage of an upcoming State Supreme

Court decision. Our state attorney general, Pam Bondi has requested a ruling on the language of the Proposition of the petition to vote for Medical Marijuana November 2014. The wording on the ballot, November 2014 Mid Term Elections, is accused of being misleading to the public.

Will the public infer that only the really suffering will be eligible for Medical Marijuana, as the conservatives favor, or will the public infer lesser suffering could be relieved, and insist on making use much more wide spread?

One anti this Medical Marijuana proposition state level government politician individual postulated this: "I want you to picture a young college student who has anxiety over exams. The student goes to the doctor. The doctor prescribes Marijuana. This isn't clear to the public that that could happen as this proposition is written." [As heard and remembered.] An NPR, National Public Radio, WGCU Ft. Myers FL covered this tax payer paid public servant saying this into a microphone for their radio audience.

The question to ask that postulating politician is "What do you know that the college student and the doctor do not know? Where are the meat and potatoes of your argument?" Indeed.

Seven hundred thousand signatures by February 2014. Five hundred thousand signatures are in place early December 2013. A court ruling is the immediate hurdle. May logic, truth and justice prevail.

Yes! the court ruled to accept the Medical Marihuana proposition as petition signed for the November 2014 mid term elections! February, 2014.

ammajjammajjammajjamma

In a Report televised April 18, 2013 of a Congressional hearing to review Eric Holder's 2014 budget for the Justice

Department: Representative Andy Harris, Republican from Maryland asked Attorney General Holder,

"In the light of the Preemptive Federal law concerning Marihuana legality, are you preparing a case against recreational Pot legalization in Colorado or Washington?"

He erroneously reminded the filled room that Marihuana is the "gateway drug" and the Federal Law must preempt state law to protect children from this danger. He, Representative Harris, was alarmed by the two states whose people legalized recreational Pot. He seemed reluctant to incarcerate over medical Marihuana as legalized by so many states.

Representative Jo Bonner, Republican from Alabama, wanted to know about Federal Marihuana arrests. He wondered out loud.

"It's either dangerous or it's miss classified as a Schedule I Drug."

Thank you. Now please work to correct the erroneous classification, Senator Bonner.

Eric Holder said he has to "prioritize resources".

okokokokokokokokokokokokokokokokokokokoko

January 2013 in a two to one decision the United States Court of Appeals for the District of Columbia Circuit Court ruled Pot must remain classified as a Schedule I drug. The reasoning: The DEA, The Federal Drug Enforcement Agency, had maintained in the case they won that the efficacy proof in their repertoire of known studies proving successful application of Marihuana as medicinal, is non existent. The District of Columbia Appeals Court accepted the Drug Enforcement Agency's case as valid. The efficacy study requirement is a Drug Enforcement Agency rule.

The court said it wasn't ruling on whether Marihuana has medicinal benefits or not, they simply agreed the paper proof of medicinal benefit wasn't on the table.

Consider that it's illegal to do a study of contra banded Pot without a permit from the Drug Enforcement Agency or the Food and Drug Administration or get a permit for a study from Federal Attorney General's office. They don't give permits because of the limitations that are in place, their rules again, on with whom and where the study may be done. High hurdles. A genuine Catch 22!!

The case was brought by ASA, Americans for Safe Access. They sued the DEA to reclassify Pot as a lesser drug than the worst classification, Schedule I. They lost, appealed and lost.

Too bad the ASA didn't have a top oncologist testifying. Would they have listened? Maybe one did testify.

In fact, since 2007 Clinical trials have proven Marijuana's ability to relieve neuropathic pain as revealed in three published reports. This from the United For Care website.

United For Care, People United for Medical Marijuana, has a petition in Florida for a Medical Marijuana proposition to be on the November 2014 midterm election ballot.

They allow:

1. People want this to pass, as shown by seven to three out of every ten surveyed.

2. Doctors may prescribe cocaine and morphine but not Marijuana. Without standing apparently is a list of diseases known as treatable with Marijuana. They are AIDS, Cancer, Glaucoma, Multiple Sclerosis, Hepatitis C, Epilepsy, Chronic Pain, and Injuries. Also Migraine Headaches and Depression. Yet in

Florida to possess Marijuana when not in private away from prying eyes is criminal.

3. Supporters are institutional, renown, huge in the American Medical world. Go to the United for Care web site.

4. Supporters are from many publications across the country. See a list of many newspaper establishment endorsements.

5. Starting nearly eighteen years ago the people of many states have passed by ballot medical Marijuana use as legal.

   In these states the seriously ill are no longer criminalized.

   {Unsung use of the Severability clause, 118 and 185, this book, when President Obama excused the nation's seriously ill as okay to use Cannabis. Perhaps?}

6. The AMA, the American Medical Association, states it believes doctors and patients should be at liberty to select the most effective treatment with out interference from the current misplaced criminality of either party, doctor or patient.

Marijuana, no overdose deaths. Many therapeutic applications. We as a people are ill served by our loss of legal access to Marijuana, a multiple application asset to the humon condition.

abcabcabcabcabcabcabcabcabc

Arthritis? Pain in general? Glaucoma? A general practitioner doctor is seen on camera interviewing and diagnosing a patient. The doctor seems to require a body of details around a long standing already in treatment condition from the patient looking for more successful relief, Cannabis. Progress, is a patient to Doctor relationship. No Progress, we are denied legality Federally.

An early nineties aired TV show, The Botany of Desire, a two decade plus old Public Broadcasting System documentary, is the referenced source of the above televised scene. It re-aired mid 2005 or so. The show has three stories each of one of the three different plants adapting to make their own evolution and planetary success progress with the help of our adaptations.

First, tulips. Tulips experienced accelerated value. A particular strain of an actually defective bulb at it's zenith being worth the cost of a house in Holland for a brief time until that bubble burst creating historical ruin in Holland. This happened some hundreds of years ago and is renown as the story of a great tulip triumph brought down by greed.

Then Cannabis. We learn about the morphing of Marihuana into a resiny behemoth under the care of true botanical genius. Once our mid to late nineteen sixties leadership had soldiers fly over Mexican Marijuana fields spraying Paraquat, poison, poison for Grass, Pot, destined for state side consumption, why, American entrepreneurs began growing, growing more and more superior strains. Thus began world wide growers so sophisticated and so outrageously hi-tech and savvy all Pot is better now.

The root cause for this quantum leap in Marijuana quality is attributed to the poisoning of Pot growing in Mexico. The United States Federal government under President Lyndon Johnson flew American planes to crop dust Pot crops in Mexico with Paraquat. American home growing of Cannabis took hold achieving excellence to save Americans from our governments deadly poisoning of crops bound for American consumption. A true American business success story albeit the sale of contraband Cannabis Herb vegetation.

The PBS, Public Broadcasting Station, TV show then tells us about the potato. We learn how the Irish Potato Famine resulted from growing only one strain of potato in Ireland. Which was fine until a disease wiped out all their potato crops practically at once. In Peru the people have a potato based diet that developed many strains of potatoes, thus side stepping famine. A Potato story of failure in one place is a triumph in another.

The commentator of the Botany of Desire PBS TV show wove the three stories together to make the point that while we are advancing we humons are also bringing winners in the plant world forward in an evolutionary march. Genetic engineering was not the big news when this show originally aired. Realize this unusual fact from history: The Dutch turned carrots from white to orange to commemorate the House of Orange in the 16th century. Therefore we eat orange carrots to this day.

acacacacacacacacacacacaca

Imagine Catsup is contraband. Would you give it up? Want to grow your own tomatoes? Not if Ketchup can be made from them. Suppose the American Medical Association spoke up and said Licopine is a valuable asset to health and Catsup is a great source. So what! Still the politicians, our legislators, hold to the easily disprovable notion that tomatoes may be poisonous. Do we quietly grow tomatoes under a full spectrum bulb in a closet? Is our defiance evidenced by eating catsup on our burgers with the shades down? Do we share with others our Catsup underworld connection for our hidden supply? Does a vast empire grow out of smuggling tomatoes into the States?

Do turf wars erupt? Of course. We really love tomatoes. A tomato substitute is produced. It will never be as good as a beautiful tasty ripe tomato but it's legal and may hurt you. Is that the America you live in?

Is ours a government that can't stop persecuting it's own taxpaying non criminal citizens? Is material greed the reason we continue decades of misery, incarceration and heartbreak of American Citizen Pot People? We are persecuted by bad law. Bad law imposed on the American people and consequently the people of the world, done erroneously and nefariously, done by including the medicinal Herb Marihuana in the Narcotics Tax Act of 1937, establishing a nefarious Drug war policy in 1970, and stupidly keeping inclusion of Cannabis as a Schedule I Felonious Possession 'Drug'. This is clearly Persecution.

What about "We hold these Truths to be self-evident, that all Mun are created equal, that they are endowed by their Creator with certain Inalienable Rights, that among these are Life, Liberty, and the Pursuit of Happiness - That to secure these Rights, Governments are instituted among Mun, deriving their just Powers from the Consent of the Governed, that whenever any Form of Government becomes destructive of these Ends, it is the Right of the People to alter or abolish it, and to institute new Government, laying its Foundation on such Principles, and organizing its Powers in such Form, as to them shall seem most likely to effect their Safety and Happiness."?

The Declaration of Independence, Action of the Second Continental Congress, July 4,1776. We've got the power.

???????????????????????????????

Congress has snuck up on us over the decades. We are no longer a free people. Not that our rights have been stripped away, no, we acquiesced. We listen to the news of others in the Marijuana supply chain getting caught. We read in the paper of another grow house discovered. We are grateful our dealer is so Podunk.

What power is this keeping us in check? Why, knowing jail and court and ruin and expense await the hapless Pot Head who sells to friends if they hit a trip wire to be caught.

Marijuana is contraband. Congress made it so. However, the people touching this vegetation cannot be summarily tried as criminal, but are. Cannabis is NOT legally criminalized. It's unconstitutionally illegal. How so? Congress may confiscate the vegetation legally and perhaps levy a fine, but may not arrest the individuals. Not only because it's unjustifiable but because Congress with the President's signature, still may not arbitrarily group innocent people as criminal. There is no legal isolating a subset of good Americans as criminal without a just cause that becomes an Amendment to the United States Constitution, a legal Prohibition. A 'drug policy' is not adequate for an American to be punished for nothing.

Standards of truth and justice are built into our evolving legislation. The slaves are free. Wemon have the vote. Marijuana possession is not a crime inside your home when not exposed to the police should you have cause to invite same into your home. Persecution describes the abuse we allow to consume individuals, families and communities over Cannabis.

It's as though Rosa Parks imagined as a legitimate Pot aficionado has to ride on the outside of the bus taking come what may with no seat, no rights, no freedom. Un-American. Shameful.

What child can make sense of a world that condones alcoholism by advertising, ubiquitous tobacco addiction, no background checks on gun ownership at the point of sale, all manner of reckless behavior on the playing field, pills to ask for at the doctor's office that the TV voice says causes death sometimes, and more.

The child hears the words Medical Marijuana many times over. Is Cannabis an asset to the humon condition? Yes.

State legal doctors prescribe Cannabis legally and freely. Nobody dies or kills. Patients improve.

Florida state legislators in Tallahassee are working to make legal a strain of Marihuana said to calm epileptic seizures in children. The strain lacks significant THC so maybe the nay sayers will back off. March 10, 2014.

How, must the child wonder, can adults be trusted when such hypocrisy, prejudice and bigotry are displayed.

Our jails overflow with non criminals. For sure it isn't Pot's fault we let Congress get away with persecution of possessors of a beneficial Herb.

A Florida State legislator got publicity for introducing a Legalize Pot bill. He expects his Republican led state legislators colleagues to keep it from a vote. March, 2014.

So why hasn't a lawyer representing a Pot possessing persecuted defendant stood up and presented all the obvious evidence supporting an individual's inalienable right to smoke or eat or possess whatever substance nature provides, especially if it's safe and promotes happiness? Fear of disbarment and ostracizing? Who knows? Maybe the Mafias and Cartels, FDA? Law Enforcement, itself?, are watching to quell any such action.

Maybe the rich and powerful are successfully lobbying and worse to destroy legalizing Pot in favor of the status quo that enriches them. Remember how significant switching from a carbon, fossil fuel, fiber to the renewable easy access non polluting Cannabis as Hemp fiber for industrial use will be toward eliminating dependency on fossil fuels.

Once Pot is sold freely and openly much ludicrously lucrative criminal activity will vanish. Cannabis possession doesn't harm a person unless arrested for same. It is quite definitely harmless in any quantity in proximity to anyone, anywhere. Weed is not contaminating, poisonous or damaging by touch or taste or ingestion or by inhaling the substance as smoked. Period. Why would we be born with THC receptors in our brains if non lethal, non addictive Cannabis were not welcomed by our minds and bodies?

Let the Pot Nay Sayers parade their rhetoric endlessly.

What is the worry? The Herb will likely never be mandatory to consume. Simply stop the heinous ignorant unlawful persecution of people over a health restoring Herb. _Such unseemly Apartheid is the Evil Root Cause of all our Woes_.

We don't know how to control our Congress to stay on track serving and protecting us legitimately. It's time we learned how.

The voting public of the states with longest term Legal Medical Marihuana have attested, and the passage of time has shown, there is no evidence to refute the judgment of these pro Pot voters arising.

Marijuana is a proven asset to the humon condition for over five thousand years of recorded history. Nothing has changed except bigotry and hypocrisy hold our country's reins.

################

Keep in mind safety and happiness are not by products of tobacco use or possession. Harvested tobacco leaves tend to initiate with a horrible rash all those who come near to the leaves for the first time. What was that movie with Elizabeth Taylor and Troy Donahue? We saw his rash. In his movie character Troy had his shirt off in a room full of cut tobacco leaves and his camera ready bare back was a mass of red welts, nickel and dime size. Good effects.

Maybe happiness ensues if one is profiting from tobacco sales.

People careless with cigarettes all too often cause fires that burn up people, houses, businesses and forests. Amazingly Pot does not. Pot goes out before igniting something else. Once legal, people may successfully substitute occasional Pot use for an otherwise unbreakable tobacco habit, thus ending their physical addiction to tobacco. Likely most useful to the recently nicotine addicted. Stop tobacco smoking and eliminate yourself from the thirty three percent of tobacco users with the statistical likelihood of a miserable death by tobacco.

When people have Marijuana to inhale or eat they opt to stay sober or more sober.

Pot users drift away from much alcohol use if not already hugely physically addicted to alcohol. Some drop cigarettes fairly easily by substituting Pot.

Picture three legitimate giant industries, Alcohol, Tobacco, and Pharmaceutical. Four, add Big Cancer.

Add most of the law enforcement community who remain ignorant of Marijuana benefits or are hypocrites, all of whom like staying employed. See all the courts and prison systems, urine test items and labs, untold armies of people working to relieve the people of the United States and the world of their access to Cannabis.

Do you see why there is no change to the status of Marijuana even in the face of the obvious truth about the good it does? By the way, in order to protect it's police force from any first hand experience or knowledge of Cannabis the Miami Police Department in the mid 'eighties' required it's applicants to state they never tried Cannabis. Sympathy and understanding based on personal experience would interfere with effectiveness, no doubt.

This is not to say law enforcement people are above enjoying Cannabis. No, hypocrisy is another by product of Pot criminalization. Sort of like married Newt Gingrich's hot and heavy pursuit of impeachment for then President Bill Clinton for his succumbing to his sexy intern's enticements. This while Newt himself had for all that time a full blown mistress he kept for years living close by. To be fair he did eventually marry her after divorcing his second wife. The crime here is that Newt got away with besmirching extremely our President. Smarmy tactics, Newt.

A certain Fox News Commentator whose initials are G.R. mentioned in his published autobiographical book that in college he was a Pot smoker. He was a Pot smoker in the early seventies, for sure. He also admitted taking Penn State college exams for others while high. His autobiography said so. They got good grades on the tests taken for them, his book said.

Our esteemed President Barrack Obama it was revealed by a spread published in Times magazine during the election run-up for the Presidency in '08, did smoke Pot rolled in a joint. Time magazine published the whole roll of film shot in his Freshmon Yale dorm room by an acquaintance. The photos show him casually toking on a joint. We see in the Time magazine article every frame shot during that one visit to his dorm room by this one acquaintance with a camera during his freshmon year. She shot him from mid chest up wearing a light color or white dress shirt, sleeves rolled up, joint pinched between his thumb and index finger, right hand. Smoke wafting.

The story included three full pages depicting every frame of the twenty four shots. He still got elected President. The article stated our 44th president stopped smoking Pot while still a Freshmon at Yale. He later graduated from Columbia University, successfully of course, and has distinguished himself honorably by becoming a Senator then our President.

Twice. President Barrack Obama won a second term.

Ron Paul, Texas United States Senator of twelve years campaigned as a Republican nomination hopeful for President. He prefers drug legalization. Ron Paul said he hopes to influence the Republican platform with his ideas at the convention in Tampa, summer 2012. Not so much it turned out.

He wants to see Pot legalized for everybody among other ideas. His son is Republican Senator Rand Paul, a Grand 'Ol Party potential Presidential contender, the 2016 election.

Five unknown Presidential contenders 2012 were given their own debate, cameras on them, on stage behind podiums. A total of twelve candidates, was it, had their names on the ballot for president. The secondary runners debate was interesting because of the two who spoke decisively that Pot must be legal.

It's apparent to all Americans we have a deep divide of opinion on the subject of legalizing Marihuana possession.

Many have incorporated anti-'drug' sentiment in their core values. Duped. Never was any 'drug' user/abuser anything but a citizen, statistically no worse or better criminally for the 'drug' used than anyone else for their preferences and as deserving of consumer protections thus making for a level playing field for comparison.

In America a proven asset to the humon condition is cause for Punishing Americans, by a contestable almost 'law'. Two top lethal drugs on the harm index pay government supporting taxes and kill lots of their consumers and lots of innocent bystanders.

Aside: Adding Industrial Hemp to our repertoire of resources can only be a positive. Think of Hemp Crete. Think of the jobs created. The DuPont Era of Petroleum dominating over all competition, over.

The most likely to harm you inadvertently drugs, prescription ones, are legal. The addicts of opiate drugs are not inherently criminal either. The issue is not a law enforcement issue at all, only one for compassion and assistance as needed. Just being legal is no endorsement.

The solution known as the Drug War has been far worse for the humon race than all the 'drugs' consumed ever could.

From the Alcohol Prohibition on, the massive illegal monetary gains made by individuals denying other individuals en masse something they want universally has been irresistible and profoundly damaging beyond comprehension to all people. It's time to let empathy and compassion rule.

.o.o.o.o.o.o.o.o.o.o.o.

Many want to enforce a 'majority rule' stance.

The approval for legal Cannabis is fifty seven percent according to Spring 2013 polls. Clearly over fifty percent of the public favor legal use of Cannabis. An under fifty percent favorable accounting can no longer be the backbone of the argument to keep the status quo.

Approval percent keeps climbing to an average of over seventy percent, all political persuasions, late December, 2013.

In fact, if even one unexceptional individual can be said to have a legitimate claim to sanctioned possession or use then anyone may have the same. We don't need the majority of us to want or believe any one thing to extend the right to any individual to believe or want to do any one thing as long as the rest of us are not harmed.

Would you ride a motorcycle to jump across a huge open space? No? Well Evil Kinevil did. He availed himself of that right and so may you. We do not provide perfect protections of our citizens from the potential of alcohol induced highway monslaughter although we easily could with a device installed as a pass/fail sobriety test in order to be allowed to start a car. That's for known drunks. Buy your own hand held alcohol detector, if you wish.

Nor do we shield ourselves from second hand tobacco smoke outside a storefront, another alterable fact by legislative and judicial agreement. Some public exterior places do boast the privilege of no cigarettes or no smoking. And the trend is growing. Municipalities are carving out smoke free properties such as library grounds and courthouse steps for it's citizens.

We the people may win at last.

odjodjodjodjodjodjodjodjodjodjdo

There is a major distinction to be made between public and private places, physical locations. Our representation is charged with making the laws that keep the public places safe. Government inspection of our homes generally stops after the original certificate of occupancy is given with code enforcement requirements met for the initial occupancy.

Our representation defines safe for us. It is not safe, but allowed, for you to breathe the second hand smoke that is a cloud you and your perhaps toddler size child must pass through to enter the mall or grocery store. Inside will be smoke free.

At present we do not allow open alcohol consumption in public anywhere. Hence the brown paper bag. The law works. Alcohol is consumed openly where licensed by the proprietor or privately. No open alcohol containers allowed in the cabin of a vehicle.

Privately: The places, locations, whose owner is not the government or leased by the government. No taxpayer money support in sight. Makes sense. Let Pot enjoy café's and clubs, home use and cultivation, all the benefits accorded beer and wine, home growing and sharing, the works! We must understand and begin protecting the rights of all citizens.

Cannabis deserves to be legal. Cannabis has been demonstrated to help maintain health. We shouldn't need a dire illness to have Pot legally. It's an asset to healthy people too.

It's scary to think of all the money, American tax payer dollars formerly paying for a Drug War, made available for other purposes once Cannabis is an ordinary commodity, especially when Pot is taxed when sold commercially. Like tomatoes, we will grow what we please, buy what's grown by others as we please. Taxing commercial sale is easily enough since tax you must.

Concentrate on truth and justice. See a new world order emerge. Trust follows Truth and Justice. Without this inevitable growth in compassion and understanding what use have we for Freedom? It is only shadowy and weak. We cannot lead the world until we begin treating our own citizenry with genuine knowledgeable respect.

The Ugly Truth about Marihuana is the shameful callousness of ongoing persecution of innocent people who are caught and arrested for possession of a God Given Natural Resource that is clearly a Health Restorative. It's also clearly true that we as a people must get this corrected in order to begin to be an honest and honorable people deserving to lead the world out of the darkness of cruel and unusual punishment of it's people.

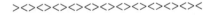

Is not Syria with it's war on it's people by a miserable dictator leader and the current state of the after math of the Arab Spring a revelation to us? How far is there to go towards a world with the ability to protect the common mon from imposed tyrannical disaster? Beyond the killing of it's own rebels and innocent population in Syria, now the warring dictator goes all the way to intimidating his own citizens with possible nerve gas bombs. This is bad. The rest of the free world will have to retaliate on behalf of the victims or not.

The nerve gas issue in Syria came and went and is back, August 2013. The civil war is on there. Egypt is in turmoil. The deposed Egyptian tyrant was replaced by a democratically elected leader who was so bad the people rose up to oust him. To get the job done the Egyptian military stepped up. So the people supporting the non-secular recently ousted president are at war to get him back as president. It's a mess, August, 2013.

How long before this idiocy is over? The rebels will win, but when? Or not?

Time has not worked a change. Months are not enough. The Arab Spring countries are left to scrap among themselves internally with their neighboring countries worrying over the millions of self exiling Fugitives from the violence. Overwhelmed, their surprised neighbors involuntarily host the Fugitives in endless camps housing the millions of homeless people.

)))))))))))))))))(((((((((((((((

The Palestinians and Israelites are skirting substantial revising because they can't find mutual respect. The Israelis won't pull back. They keep building in the Gaza.

The Palestinians can't muster enough muscle in global popular opinion to force their right to a land of their own.

So they war on. Secretary of State Kerry is doing his job.

Each has conceded an inch.

Palestinians are gaining the hearts and minds to embrace there plight. February 2014.

Syria is still warring, end of March 2014. The dictator a non performer regarding his United Nations agreement. Some chemicals have been handed over.

Iran and North Korea are working together on their rocket science, still a long way from arming anything with a nuclear warhead. North Korea did a successful four stage rocket launch. Observed wobbling of the rocket negated fears of an impending aggression catastrophe, 2013?

China and India are bright spots of economic growth again. The Euro zone is post recession, barely. We've steadied up. Late August 2013 the economic picture overall looks improved and improving. Wobbly maybe.

ooooooooooooooooooooooooooooo

Worldwide we mourned the deaths of twenty little children, December 15, 2012, because a young male, aged twenty, entered a school with enough weaponry to very quickly off twenty first grade aged children and six adults at the school. He'd already killed his mother at home in her bed. He killed himself at the scene. The entire massacre took place in well under five minutes, he was so armed with automatic clips of bullets and guns.

peacepeacepeacepeacepeacepeacep

Leading the free world to keep it free and to help others overcome oppression worldwide is a tall order these days.

Don't be afraid. When we are standing up for each other's rights we are our strongest. Imagine yourself as Rosa Parks. You sit down in the vacant seat in the first half of the bus. You are arrested. You, in the case of a Marihuana possession arrest, hold a press conference to protest the lack of truth and justice. You are armed with the Truth.

<u>You want the right to board the bus</u>. You seek Justice. At some point will come the tipping point and just like the long awaited and still fought for total equality for other minority rights you are in a minority that deserves the freedom to pursue happiness unhampered by another's mere ignorance.

No excuses. Freedom is your right. Protective laws aplenty are in place that apply equally to everyone.

No worries, there's no new breed of criminal.

We are told eight percent of Americans imbibe Pot.

Approximately twenty eight million of us from a census survey, 2011?

You courageously write a letter to your Congresspersons saying you want Cannabis to be legal in this country. Refuse to accept without comment the arrest put in your local paper of a person thrown into the criminal justice system as a supposed benefit to the rest of us over a misdemeanor trace amount of Marihuana along with a felony charge for whatever paraphernalia, for example. This is upsurd. Let everyone you know know that you are ashamed that we are denying the truth about Cannabis. Justice is not served when the innocent are preyed upon by taxpayer supported bad law enforcement. We deserve aware legislation, not incarceration.

Even if you want the police to continue the activities of their useless expensive posturing and citizen persecution to rid us of contraband, gambling and prostitution, no one can make a legitimate case for keeping Pot contraband. It's the tax free inflated profits from Contraband Market dealing that makes users of the hard drugs proliferate.

Because prescription drug pain killers are the foremost abused drugs of choice in our country, the former hard drugs being passed over, to surge again, the profits of Marihuana sales sometimes carry financially the old line of hard drugs.

This told on camera by an officer taped burning pot grown on public land in South Carolina. It aired in the Botany of Desire show aired on the Public Broadcasting System initially some years ago.

Great Show, three stories. One told the amazing rise of value of exotic tulip bulbs in Holland about three hundred years ago. One bulb equaled the same value as a house. The bubble burst. In Ireland only one variety of potato is planted. Enter a potato disease that wipes out that variety.

Killer famine resulted.

The third story, Pot plants are sprayed with poison while growing in Mexico for our market. Soon local commercial grow houses attract geniuses to promulgate a quantum leap of quality, resinous Pot for the American market. Three Flora interacting with humons with outcomes that enrich the variety and depth of their genetic strains outrageously.

Amazing tulips, potato varieties super promulgated, the same for Cannabis, all as though the plants maximized themselves through us by desire, the Botany of Desire.

############

Okay, now you may be afraid. The Sequester has been in place since March 1, 2013. For more heartbreak, the Government is shut down on the Federal level. Only the essential personnel remain at work on October 8, 2013. President Obama addresses the country to make clear that the week just spent with a partial, really mostly, shut down of the Federal Government has hurt our country as a whole and Americans as individuals. It's a paid vacation for furloughed Federal employees. Congress passed keeping furloughed Federal employees' paychecks as exempt.

The impending deadline, October 17th 2013, for Congress to raise the debt ceiling to pay the Federal Government's bills on time, is in peril of being ignored. Our government defaulting on debt payment, a true failure, mucking up any hope of avoidance of a downturn economically, likely worldwide. It's a weak moment for our reserves to fill in a gap were there a defaulting of the United States Treasury even if a brief number of days. There is no net until we fabricate it from more borrowing abroad.

Unappetizing.

No, it's a revolting development just to be at day nine of a Federal Government shutdown with eight days to go to an end to the Standoff that requires the GOP side to back off the shutdown and the government bill paying default. The Grand Old Party Republicans are saying ad nauseum something like, unless we, the Republicans, get a concession of something as yet unspecified unless it's Postpone The Affordable Care Act funding which is, we know, off the table.

Two days to go and counting, October 15, 2013, the United States Government is fifteen days mostly Shut Down, causing ripples of ruin in American lives. The debt ceiling itself is up in two days, raising renewal to cover bills not paid not yet addressed by our United States Congress, due to Tea Party presumptions and poor, horrific, choices made by House Majority Leader Representative Boehner. We face the unheard of Threat of Default with global repercussions if not settled immediately. We appear incompetent by threatening failing.

Since we are experiencing the GOP's request to de-fund Obama Care, in part now, President Obama is gathering Congressmun to help put the brakes on a further debacle.

Stay tuned. Obama Care left the table to seep back. The few who are Tea Party are weighty, we know not why. Perhaps because the participating bottom rung Tea Party enthusiasts are attracted by the less government rhetoric unaware of the United States governments inextricable role in the well being of so much, being gone would be enough to burst their complacent still comfortable middle class life looking to pay less for their taken for granted good portions unable to understand how America thrives on the well fed and educated from all walks of life. We see decisions made to keep a congressional seat over keeping our American collective Life's Future out of jeopardy.

"Money talks, nobody walks." Classic wheeler dealer line.

ZVZVZVZVZVZVZVZVZVZVZVZ

April 1, 2014 we are treated to an example of the future should the contemporary Republican side of the House of Representatives have it's leadership's way. The wealthy will have even greater wealth. Americans benefiting from their Social Security secured Medicare, Medicaid, Food Money, become productive with subsidized Education and such. Infrastructure top-notch, or any other important underpinning of our society should be better than it is this day as is appropriate for the prosperity abundant in our country, not deprived.

One can only suppose the family of the author of this silly projected ten year U.S. of A. budget as unveiled would be expected to have his children go without shoes so Daddy could have a new tie.

The timing for this budget plan and transparent appeal to the wealthy like minded? A pitch for personal funding, plain and simple. You shall remain nameless.

OhOhOhOhOhOhOhOhOhOh

Are you guilty of supporting the illegal Contraband Markets by keeping them illegal?

We learned this from a man on the front lines of Marijuana plant eradication: Again, Marijuana is the cash machine that often supports all the other not always profitable hard drug sales. Marijuana, by being illegal, is keeping the hard drugs available by underwriting that arm of the illicit drug trade by turns, in effect. A renewed cocaine market is exporting to Australia and on to China and points in between.

Sounds like we will be extraordinarily culturally better off with legalization of Pot, doesn't it?

Meet a South Carolina Police Officer, a law enforcement team leader in west South Carolina interviewed on camera for the PBS TV show The Botany of Desire explaining the task of removing and burning(!) the Cannabis vegetation he and his team find, year in and year out. The large plantings are gone, we are told. There's more in smaller patches and the Pot plants are elusively located. The show may have been aired originally in the '90's. Years ago it aired on the Public Broadcasting Station, WEDU, Miami, FL.

The show's segment on Cannabis finished with us watching the four or five South Carolina cops monning a small haystack size bonfire of Pot, thick smoke filling the air. The men stayed busy a few feet away, busy with the fire, wearing police uniforms. Burning out in the open, smoke billowing away, is their usual method of disposal for Marihuana. . . . No kidding.

There is now a United States Congressional law describing proper disposal of Pot since 2010, see Acts of Congress reference 'drugs' list, without elaboration, #2 page 80, this book.

Once again the specter of Cannabis as the bridge or Gateway Drug emerges. Yes, the truth of this is not much of the whole story, though.

But Yes, if the person who gave you your first Pot or so turns out to be a store of illicit drugs on two feet and you offer little or no resistance, you are likely 'Done from the Git Go'.

Naturally the gateway, the bridge is best disappeared and quick. Only one way. From contraband to Free Market Commodity overnight. Instant success with thoughtful legalization of Marijuana. No further connection to lawlessness to exist. Like Catsup.

Serve and Protect. The whole Justice Department top to bottom is there to take care of we citizens by serving and protecting.

Our Legislative branch top to bottom is charged with making and amending the laws that are subsequently enforced as the service and protection. Congress also funds or not.

In their turn our courts discover the guilt or innocence of the justly accused or make relatively final who may do what, where & when, and possibly, how.

Public servants, your attention, please. Here is the dilemma regarding Contra banded Marijuana, a Schedule I Drug, as it continues to share this worst 'drug' tier with cocaine and heroin in our judicial system. Worst means the harshest sentencing. The law covers possession unconsumed. It administers severity of guilt by the weight of the said contraband. Before disposal Pot Plants are counted and weighed dirt and all, we hear. Dirt too? Could that be?

Recently found huge acreages are planted with Pot on public lands we are told. Actually inside our State and National Parks! 2012.

2013, a seventy six year old war on Pot has continued since the Marihuana Tax Act in of 1937, four years past the United States Constitutional Amendment ending the Prohibition Against Alcohol by Congressional repeal in 1933.

In 1914 the Harrison Act Criminalized the opiates. Pot was added as a contraband narcotic in the Narcotic Tax Act of 1937. The Drug War gained traction with the creation of it's own department during Nixon's administration.

Currently the Drug War is in service to the Drug Abuse Prevention Act-1970 and all it's thirty six Acts and statements.

Obvious point: the mere presence of the healing herb Cannabis which appears as vegetation in and of itself poses no threat to the possessor. Historically Marijuana held prominent place as a land erosion stopper as late as last century because it grows like a weed sending roots down very deep quickly, about twelve feet down in a year. The rope you may buy at the hardware store may be Hemp. Hemp is the common name of the non psycho active varieties. President George Washington grew it. Our government grew it out west for World War I use as rope, circa 1917.

Pot does have a rather distinct pungent aroma growing, dried for tea, cooked into oil, served in a brownie, or fired up in a pipe. Heat releases the THC. Use a water pipe or bong if you dare. Maybe it's better to inhale the medicinal smoke cooled.

Law enforcement relies on trained dogs to ferret out contraband by smell. Possession of Marihuana poses one real and every day danger. Don't get caught. Unless you are able to secure a really good lawyer you are grist for the mill.

Your opportunity to make your case before a jury is not ensured. Anyway, juries are restricted to those who will guarantee the verdict of guilty by matching only what is stated by law enforcement as fact and the letter of the law as stated by the judge. These directions are to be followed without exception so says the judge. Formulas are used to determine the punishment.

Truth: Juries have the power, once the Judge gives the case to them, to decide their verdict, no matter what's been said by the judge.

Our courts have choked off entirely the basic design of the system. Juries rule. Judges are to advise jurors. Juries once were made aware that once they have the case their deliberation may return a judgment on the law itself. Juries may Nullify.

This is a healthy part of our criminal justice system.

We would not be so far along in the systemic persecution of the people who are the end consumer of the health restorative herb, Cannabis, without the suppression of the truth about Cannabis and the open oppression of jurors. For decades jurors have been inhibited from giving their input to our evolving laws.

The facts that exonerate Marihuana are mountainous and unrelenting. Twenty states and the District of Columbia have legalized medical Marijuana as best they could. Millions upon millions of people and dollars are involved. The only danger is still the law against Pot which supports and sustains the contraband market causing so much misery daily. Once an individual is caught they become part of the penal system. A round robin of punishment ensues. The gangs and cartels are left to thrive as members rotate in and out. No gain is ever made for the public at large.

Law enforcement has yet to make a real dent in the trafficking, no contest. It's the illegality that makes the contraband market so lucrative for all three, big and little traffickers and their would be nemesis, law enforcement.

Cccccccccccccccccccccccccc

Let's examine the vegetation Cannabis as consumed. At present the Federal Government admits that those who are really sick with HIV, bad Cancer issues, etc., these people are exempt from the long arm of the law, per this current administration. For now, those having these woes may consume this gentle healer and comforter as needed without worrying they will be busted. It's obvious the truly ill are better off with Cannabis to any and all observers. Yet they must worry about the safety of the person who provides their stash. If they become strong enough maybe they could grow their own Cannabis. Is this safe too?

A prescription for Pot in the nineteen seventies, meant a suggested smoking of a basic joint every two hours, making five joints a day. Twenty eight grams to an ounce of Pot and about twenty joints from an ounce of un-cleaned Pot. In 2013 that would likely stretch to thirty joints because pot has more resin and comes cleaner. Resin is where the active ingredient THC is.

This amount would maintain a Cannabinol level for a patient. This was the norm in the early seventies. Pot with more resin, THC, means less of an amount. A little goes a long way.

nmnmnmnmnmnmnmnmnmnmnmnmnmnmnmn

Science has been shut down concerning Marijuana. No one may study for Scientific findings pro or con. No studies are done because it's contraband. Only some miniscule few have been granted a permit to study Pot ever. That permit comes from the DEA or FDA or the Federal Attorney General.

April 18th, 2013, C-Span taped a Senate hearing with Attorney General Eric Holder concerning the Budget for the Justice Department year 2014. Republican Senator Andy Harris of Maryland asked this: Because Federal law supersedes state law, why aren't the Feds bearing down on the two states working to implement Legal Recreational Pot as passed last November? "Bearing down" he said. The Senator gave the broad stroke rational of Pot as the Gateway Drug for children and that a study he did not name has shown very young children have brain aberrations of some unmentioned sort that never go away after exposure to Pot. News not widely known appearing blatantly over inflated at best, if remotely true. Study results also appear to lack any implicit negative outcome, could be a brain upgrade.

Attorney General Holder answered ultimately that he would continue to mitigate the problem of 'drug' abuse with the application of resources as best allocated in these times of budget restraint and subsequent prioritizing. Another Republican Senator, Jo Bonner, said the danger he associates with Schedule I classification should make it a priority. Then he added, "If it's properly classified as Schedule I."

Improperly classified, yes. Yet somehow, no change on the horizon.

Note: January 2013, A District of Columbia Circuit Court Appeal to reclassify Pot to a II, III, IV, or V Scheduled Drug, anything but the horrific erroneous Schedule I, failed. The DEA won again. The DEA had no study to prove Medical

Marihuana efficacy, is why. Two of the three judges on the Circuit agreed with the first ruling.

****

The end consumer experiences mood elevation that is mostly subtle. Talk-a-tive-ness may ensue. Need vigor? You got it. Need to relax? You got it. Social unease? Mitigated. Pleasure in food, dancing, lovemaking, working, playing, et.al. may become more focused. Laughter comes more easily and freely, depending on the individual and circumstances. People use Pot because it's good for people, unequivocally. There is no lethal dose. Caffeine has a lethal dose.

Literal possession of Pot in your pocket or car trunk? Could be trouble with the law. Note: Keep your hands washed. Sniffer dogs smell door handles of cars and knobs of doors.

Actual post consumption state of the user? Virtually undetectable. No measure of intoxication is possible because Marihuana contains no toxins. No measure of impairment is available for the reason no impairment of eye hand coordination or reaction time takes place, on the contrary.

Plus, anger is not a by product, a' contraire. Twelve Reefer Madness genru movies came out in the 1930's rolling out the first big wave of demonization. Big Pharmaceuticals, example Pfizer, produced a smear campaign. Pfizer was introducing their patented Bayer Aspirin and wanted to corner the entry level pain killer and fever reducer market.

Obdoobdobdobdobdobdobdo

The story of the Ybor City sensational and horrific massacre of the Licata Family in 1933 by an individual whose mental challenges were fully documented, served erroneously to make Marijuana illegal. The then Narcotics Bureau head, a Mr. Anslinger, crusaded hard with two hundred faked anecdotes of individuals crazed by Cannabis. The Licata Family Killer was the featured homicidal maniac. He was literally deranged. He did the massacre or was he framed? Anslinger lied blaming Marijuana. He sighted Marijuana used by the killer to be the cause to further the demonization across the finish line. Congress enacted the Narcotics Tax Act of 1937 adding Cannabis to the list of 'drugs' at the last minute.

Marijuana was included in the Narcotics Tax Act of 1937 because of Anslinger's influence. No one knows for sure why Anslinger lied. He was chummy with the DuPonts, who, like the pharmaceutical empire, wished to eliminate competition from Hemp grown to be the manufacturing fiber resource of choice in American industry. DuPont's business competition companies preferred Hemp for their fiber. The DuPont's won. Goodbye natural fiber, hello synthetic fiber for industry as a monopoly based on petroleum plastics, or fibers. Enter the Dupont Petroleum Era.

Henry Ford made a car using Hemp. Check it out.

Non-Psycho active Hemp is legally grown for export in Canada, not in America. Hemp-Crete is a worthy building material unavailable in America.

Legal Pot denial is an ugly story. It looks like manipulation of our government for private gain, screw the people, has been institutionalized since the Alcohol Prohibition. Thriving manipulation.

$$$$$$$$$$$$$$$$$$$$$$$$$$$$$$

Failure to serve and protect Cannabis consumers and their right to legally consume a vegetation that is a Creation Given Natural Resource Health Restorative and Superior Libation is obstinacy in light of the facts surrounding the Herb in question. Pot is clearly intended to restore health in the humon mind and body. This revelation trumps the lies of the nefarious greedy who are perpetuating the myth of a deterring down side to use or possession.

The criminalization of Pot is what hurts. There is no crash after the high. The wearing off is literally imperceptible to the user.

Maintaining a Cannabinol level is the perhaps superior equivalent to sustaining an even pharmaceutical presence in a humon body using a lab drug with many potentially dangerous side effects possible due to the lab drug toxins ubiquitous in boxed and bottled medications that are dangerous for humons to ingest.

No physical addiction to Marijuana is possible.

Coffee and Soda contain an additive drug, caffeine. Caffeine is used endlessly by the multitudes, many blissfully addicted. There is a lethal dose amount for the same drug caffeine that is the caffeine in our coffee and Soda Pop, by the way. And like everything else, coffee is not for everyone.

%@%@%@%@%@%@%@%@%@%@%

The obesity epidemic may well have one insidious culprit, caffeinated soda. Available everywhere, consumed preferentially, caffeinated soda is purchased as the drink of choice at the fast food restaurants and to drink at home.

Iced tea has caffeine too.

Customers are addicted to the caffeine and must return for their caffeine fix and incidentally to consume the fat filled processed foods that are popular washed down with the customers required daily stimulant that is a physiological addiction, caffeine.

mkhmkhmkhmkhmkhmkhmkhmkhmkh

It is up to individuals to speak up with the truth about Marihuana when possible. Inevitably we will embrace Marihuana as the panacea to solve outrageous health care costs. Turns out with the stress of illegality removed from Marihuana possession, casual use nets individuals quick recuperation at the onset of an illness. It's crazy, but who knows, could be Pot prevents or cures cancer or both. We deserve to find out. It surely looks like Pot does boost the immune system.

One well funded scientist has worked through to a positive result of some sort with mice using THC against cancer. So who knows?

Let's pay our law enforcement to serve and protect us, for real. Let's make Congress aware of the over whelming evidence.

Meanwhile, we are barbarians on a witch hunt attempting by persecution of the many to then prosecute the few, in too large a number, to keep misshapen and truncated the rights of the many by the intimidation. If lawmakers want respect they must start by respecting We the People. No more turning your backs on truth legislators, no more.

We the People, including Pot Aficionados, matter the most, and we want our service and protection and we want it now.

>>>>>>>>>>>>>>>>>>*<<<<<<<<<<<<<<<<<<<<<

Jews in Nazi Germany had no means to demand their government show a just cause to arrest them.

Here in America, we Potheads demand our government prove the premise behind jailing Potheads as sound, for it is a false premise. There is no way to show just cause for relieving Potheads of their liberty. There is no Amendment to our constitution to legally make such an innocent person criminal.

The public is not served or protected by this evil discrimination. Nay, we are denied legal acquisition of Pot, a proven means to our own betterment, so say more than twenty eight million Americans, eight percent of the three hundred fifty million of us.

Eight percent is the percent of our total population said to use Pot. This from a survey done by the United States government since 2010. It's believable.

Suppose this new world view is correct. The view that the people count votes, one person, one vote. Money may not vote. Imagine Leaders cultivated from the general population. Opportunities to do real good easily taken up.

Meanwhile Americans continue supporting with their taxes the notorious Drug War. The Drug War is having a centennial anniversary 2014. The Drug War in essence has one hundred years of existence February 8, 2014, beginning with President's Woodrow Wilson's signature on the Harrison Act of 1914.

By supporting contraband enforcement, we ensure ourselves a lucrative underworld contraband market. The underworld has commanded the illicit drug market including Marihuana for the seventy seven years since the Narcotics Tax Act passed Congress in 1937, this being 2014. Possession of contraband became a Federal offence if not officially purchased with the tax paid. This demonizing of a Creation Given Natural Resource Health Restorative and Superior Libation makes BIG Business the clear winner. Can you say Status Quo?

When a product is introduced to a foreign market as a western import there to modernize the buying public it is advertised. Ads show how much better the new western product is than the more primitive current solution. An example: Kotex feminine protection pads sold prefab in a box are replacing rolls of cotton at the local Pharmacia, meaning Drug Store. Okay.

Replacing the criminalized, possibly superior medicinal herb, with potentially lethal laboratory pills and encapsulated powders in the marketplace is pure evil. The marketplace is the place to compete, not subvert by control and manipulation of legislators so the good medicinal herb and superior libation can't be legally purchased.

We pay for this giant circle of victimization of ourselves.

We fill our prisons to overflow. We build more prisons. Seventy percent of all the inmates were and are in for 'drug' related convictions. Currently prisons are mandated to shrink populations such are the ongoing inhumone conditions in many prisons, for example, in California. One solution is to ship the prisoners where the accommodations are across state lines. For instance, one region has a low occupancy rate in a newly built prison. Felonious inmates are imported from too full prisons to the unoccupied prison accommodations.

Have we not endorsed this cultural norm? The Regan years, had the children's "Just Say No" campaign. How to accept Cannabis is a problem when the magnitude of the problem developed out of Cannabis being excluded from lawful behavior at purchase? Illegal Pot possession, the crime of owning a "controlled substance". Those two words together are laughable. Not only has the Illegal Drug Trade flourished, the biggest winners run countries and conduct open turf wars killing innocent bystanders exactly as the Alcohol Prohibition did. The Drug War has headlined locally across our nation as recently as this year, 2014.

One Mexican came to rule the illicit drug trade basing his empire in Chicago, Illinois. He made money going and coming, financing, importing and selling 'drugs', plus money laundering. He controlled a swath of America, all the middle third of the continental United States. He was apprehended in Mexico in March, 2014, and extradited immediately to America because the jails in Mexico are not secure for this hombre, he has so much power over so many. He escaped easily when last arrested. A Mr. Gomez by name, cartel boss extraordinaire.

Expect no change in the business model Mr. Gomez has had in place more than a decade.

Our American and multi national illegal drug entrepreneurs went High Tech and smoothed out their pipelines with more sophisticated efforts like doing massive planting of Pot plants in our huge national parks.

The point is our complicity. How is all this mammoth untaxed illicit yet just profiteering remaining illicit when the biggest population bubble before the millennials, the post World War II baby boomers, partook of Marihuana universally virtually? So many of us have first hand experience of the "harmlessness" of the no crash "high". And it's NOT physically addictive unlike routine use of the drug caffeine in coffee, tea and soda which commonly produces a physical addiction with evident withdrawal symptoms.

How does Federal legalization of Cannabis remain elusive in the face of some people enjoying state legal medical Marihuana for years and years in twenty states and soon even The District of Columbia. State level legality only. Pot remains vulnerable Federally.

"Harmless" is a lost term because of the stigma and the pre-employment pee test THC makes you fail. There are actual arrests of a million plus people a year nationally for Pot. Add the resulting negative life impact of being fed into our, so unjust on this, Criminal Justice System. Persecution over Cannabis makes victims of innocent people.

Once you are out on probation from any arrest or incarceration you report to your probation officer routinely to do a pee test you must pass controlled substance free or go to jail in hand cuffs. Fail the pee test and in moments you are on your way back to lockup, all liberty lost.

It may take as long as six months to clear one's pee for THC testing. All toxic substances are dumped very quickly by the body. Only days for alcohol or cocaine. The body stores and treasures THC. We are all born with receptors in our brains for THC. THC receptors occur naturally in our brains in several sites. We grow receptors for caffeine.

The positive for THC pee test does not qualify as criminal if you are not in the criminal justice system already. Attempt to be employed with a pee test hurdle you fail, simply no job. No legal repercussions to ensue known.

bbbbbbbbbbbbbbbbbbbbbbbbop

Depravation of Cannabis enjoyment has no beneficial or positive side effects. It's un-American to have a Cannabis demonizing law that serves to keep individuals divided and separated and fearful. Both the users and non users are kept fearful. We the people are the non winners in the Drug War.

This and so much more pain is inflicted on Americans and people through out the world at our 'drug' law policy behest. Harm that is beyond monumental. The most painful truth is law enforcement officers failing us by not informing or not being heard by their superiors when they knew Marihuana users pose no risk to others or themselves and do not go through any detoxification or withdrawal process when without their "drug of choice". Pot has about four hundred twelve ingredients, none toxic. No physical addiction possible. Good substance, meant as panacea to many, is this ancient historically respected medicinal Herb.

Back to the point. In the face of all such obvious reasons to behave sensibly, why not? We humons, we Americans and indeed, all the world's citizens are no better and no worse than the Good Germans who were not Jewish who accepted the premise of Aryan supremacy. Details never came up. That lockstep march mindset was orchestrated and dictated, and became an accomplished fact of literal mass murdering dominance.

The pre-Holocaust. Political correctness at it's worst. Evidently we, no group of humons, is above that loss of individualism and compassion for the excluded other.

In our free country even one person may choose a singular path. For example, Evil Kinevil. He set up and ran full speed up and over a huge chasm on his motorcycle aiming to defy death to accomplish the unique feat of flying so very far through the air astride a near ton of fired up metal to land safely or not on the other side. No law against that and rightfully so. A majority of us do not have to endorse another's choices.

Science should be allowed to find out factual answers to the question of just how wonderful is this unpatentable inexpensive Weed, also known as a Herb used as medicine and libation.

KKKKKKKKKKKKKKKKKKKKKKKKKKKKK

My paternal Grandfather lived with us a short while. He'd give me a nickel at age five as reward for 'pulling' him up out of his chair. He was blind and used a cane. I figured he looked a lot like my storybook Humpty Dumpty character with his smooth round belly, pants rising well up high to cover his ample belly. The pants had those spidery suspenders.

Granddaddy Hall went blind with Glaucoma. Regrettably, he didn't stay with us long at all. Later when I discovered Marihuana prevents Glaucoma, you could say I was sold.

If you are not persuaded to raise your voice making audible the necessity for our United States Congress to stop supporting the underworld's Contraband Markets, answer this: Are you so superior to me, who chooses to maintain my Cannabinol level as an asset and lives an average normal life for decades on end doing so, or am I so inferior to you for the same reason, that I should be led away in handcuffs? Punished? Persecuted? Prosecuted? Lose my liberty? Pay for the humiliation, probation, court cost, suffer, lose life momentum and become the reason for all that taxpayer overhead. No way.

Maintaining one's cannabinol level is a personal matter.

Could it be jobs, no, shareholder profits, matter more than people? Is this the same old game, get rid of the competition?

Jobs will abound if our status quo mega industries are nimble enough to switch away from the uniform practices of the day to embracing inclusiveness, meaning the creative input of all comers with the chops whether it's an innovation or the person innovating.

Jobs will migrate to regulatory work as Cannabis finally has all the respect currently accorded alcohol and tobacco with one difference: Perhaps there will be No Smoking on Public property of any sort including all roads, sidewalks, parks. Maybe in smoking booths like phone booths if the technology ever exists. Vapor delivery devices may serve for nicotine or THC.

The Pharmaceutical Empire values profits and hates competition as much now as when it produced the twelve Reefer Madness genre movies for wide distribution over eighty years ago. You may easily name ten industries that depend on Cannabis criminalization which excludes so many people arbitrarily and erroneously from lawfulness.

Example, the drug test makers. An obvious industry to likely evolve into greater wealth by discovering a new popular use for their product design with just a little imagination.

ncncncncncncncncncncn

Stop Demand? Maybe, but why? Eradicate at the source? Hasn't worked yet. Decrease the amount of controlled substances trafficked? No progress made. Demonstrably illegal drug use falls per capata when tolerance is in place. Remember, too, anyone committing any crime where a perpetrator actually criminally interacts with another's person or property, even at work, is amply covered by existing non 'drug' related law which serves to snare both the user and non user criminals. Nes pa?

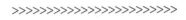

HUMON RIGHTS ABUSE

Occupy Wall Street. All around the world a great hue and cry is going out to right the wrong of lost income, work and good futures, lost in the twinkle of a decade.

Like the Big Finish Crescendo before the next roar of crashing wave, Big Business made a raid on the Cookie Jar of Common Wealth. The greedy raiding again and again until licking up every crumb of our common wealth.

The scarfing up of the last crumb of our common wealth by the greedy is the equivalent of taking our 'vehicular' ship of state, America, out for a spin and leaving her wrapped around a proverbial tree, totaled. Big Business Bankers casually getting out unscathed, tossing the keys aside and moving on to the international vehicle for a another fast ride.

To know 'how far a field' the lending institutions went away from good practices one has only to experience borrowing post Mortgage debacle lending/borrowing. The current over correction in lending, stringent entirely, works for the big institutions well because of the free money the bond market receives as seventy five BILLION dollar infusions meant as loan underwriting from the Federal Reserves monthly.

All the Bank owed property taken in foreclosure or counted as collectible debt if short of foreclosure is a plus in their asset column. Banks pay zero percent to borrow, still. March, 2014.

It's well documented how this taking of the 'reigns' by Big Business took place for good and always. The Prohibition. Making alcohol illegal made the lawless the richest in the land. The wealthiest choose our ethics by making our laws. For example, they elect those endorsing keeping contraband contraband. Since the Alcohol Prohibition contraband lawlessness produced a new dimension of the extraordinary power of ill gotten gains. The super rich attempt to make our laws suit them from behind the scene.

We individuals wrestle along sweating and confined by every Supreme Court ruling that slaps us, the we in we the people, back down. Corporations gain footholds, incursions, into humun rights and are set to oppress individual employees by virtue of corporations newly acquired status of personhood. A case in point before the Supreme Court concerns whether a private employer can drop contraception coverage from individual enployees health care insurance coverage. The Affordable Care Act says to provide same.

Once we are back on track implementing the universal acknowledgement that the individual is paramount all our relationships with government will improve dramatically.

goodbad.badgood.goodbad

We dodge the crossfire of 113th lost cause United States Congress and wonder how long we've got.

We decry the perceived ineptitude of a ham strung Administration. The Presidency itself is under siege and surviving with elegance but only as ooze finding it's way around an iron fist of media manipulation keeping so much of the population stupid, told what to believe by a single corporate entity, with an agenda. Veiled reference to Fox News Television. The tirade? Obama is the anti-you president. How Tiresome.

Second term President Obama was fairing better until the leverage of not raising the debt ceiling became the oppositions inane clout. The Republican led House of Representatives is squaring off on the public due to a faction in their ranks saying accept de-funding ObamaCare or face our Federal Government shut down for lack of funding, with a generous topping off of distain for the American public, also refusing to pay incurred debt bills. No debt ceiling raising.

The mostly all of our Federal Government Shut Down lasted sixteen days. At the eve of the seventeenth day, default on our debt payments began at midnight. The House Side of Congress was allowed to vote, at last, with naturally plenty of votes to open up the government. Furloughed federal employees could go back to work the morning of the seventeenth of October, 2013.

We are told we are not the investment risk we once were... again. The United States Government has a higher interest payment to pay on debt, must weather a drop in Gross National Product Growth by a chunk, predicted. Also are the thousands upon thousands of Americans inconvenienced by deferred pay, or no pay, or shut doors at destinations from monuments to hot dog stands.

Obama represents us as a peoples' president facing up to those greedy for control. The gluttonous media moguls and conservative demagogues, ultra wealthy types, are all wanting to keep or acquire full say over which energy sources, our armies' priorities, how security is best maintained and especially whose decisions are these. Big business, the status quo types, like money funneling up enriching the rich. Big business continues to fight for the right to be the "deciders" for these issues.

The bright future big business is angling for keeps out immigrants who work illegally. Strips government funded education from all ages of people from pre kindergarten to doctorates, at least those without familial wealth. Consolidates good paying jobs into the few and grows a cheap labor force.

Currently the sequester cuts take food from children.

During the sixteen day Federal Government shut down private and state coffers opened to fill some dire gaps.

Should government spending slow to a trickle the care of the old will be the responsibility of the young. Why not continue to have care of the old as a shared anticipated need that benefits us all eventually, care as the rightful fruition for growing old in America. Living in a free and prosperous country could and should mean reasonable care for the very young and the very old or infirm.

Vintage people evolve to emerge as surprise winners, mental and physical abilities prolonged. Prediction.

We are a country made prosperous by paying a portion of our earnings to the government and getting infrastructure, education and services back. Add Social Security Benefits and Medicare and Medicaid health care. Enter the retiring Baby Boomers. It is to our advantage to let Pot flow freely to those interested. No mandated usage. Over time it's possible we will see a reduction in the progression of common illnesses into debilitation. Perhaps Pot improves immunity protections. Lots of us will avoid the onset of illness in the first place.

Could Pot veer us away from a potential Health Care cost fiasco? With Pot legal we would save so much expense in The Judicial Branch and in the Congress. Shrinking government by applying justice and truth so actual living beings become the productive contributing souls they are meant to be? It's a Win! Win! Win! The Freed, Taxpayers, Budgets.

Perhaps all the folderol around such basic Congressional to dos as budgets and debt ceilings is a smoke screen. Smoke screens are unproductive tangents meant to keep meaningful legislation in Congress from ever being heard.

We pay for all those Congressional committees and Judicial Courts to have ourselves well looked after as we see fit. But are we well looked after? Denied legal THC at the least and suffering crushed momentum by the threat of prison, prison sentences and probation. All behind the unsupportable discrimination against our THC providers? THC is the wonderful beneficial ingredient in a health restorative Weed, for goodness sakes.

Big business believed it had to keep THC away from mainstream consumers as much as possible. The loss of any market share to Pot was not to be tolerated.

We are molded as consumers. Legislation steers us.

Are we not still using fossil fuels and seeking natural gas from fracking? Against all logic for decades we keep on course - we make war, we build arsenals, we let our people pay the price in blood and treasure and most of us know we are manipulated for ill.

Solar energy capture could have been the next greatest employer and fuel source for decades already if our leaders had so deemed.

Late is still better than never......

The most heinous humon rights abuse is the one written as law. The Nazis had only to make Jews illegal to gain the upper hand to bring about such a dreadful conclusion. We understand the majority is vulnerable to such persuasion. Acceptance of the unthinkable. Extermination of the undesirable. Vermin to rid the world of lest contamination occur. Never again we said.

The Aryan Supremacy has to be protected from the risk of contamination of it's bloodlines. This is not a past tense endeavor. White race supremacy is alive and well. Christian morality seen through a supremacist eyes sees separation and legal oppression and criminalization as reliable tools for preventing the contamination by proximity that could ultimately corrupt the supremacist bloodlines.

Big Money and Big Oppression are United.

Look now at the making contraband of 'drugs'.

The United States Congress that passed the Narcotics Tax Act of 1937 was singularly corrupt. The congressmen were bought and paid for by the former alcohol bootleggers seeking the return of a lucrative contraband market. Marihuana was added to the Act at the last minute.

The only organized group to protest and so quickly? The American Medical Association. Implementation of the Narcotics Tax Act of 1937 meant setting about to control groups of minorities; Blacks, People of Color, Latinas and Latinos, Hispanics, and Asians are exclusively those arrested. This exclusive discrimination lasted the first thirty years past becoming 'law'. By the nineteen seventies persecuted ranks were swollen to include the young adult Baby Boomers, the hippies. The draft for the Vietnam War snared our best and brightest.

History reveals the demonization of Pot was orchestrated by one man with the ear of Congress. One man named Henry Anslinger, head of the Federal Bureau of Narcotics in the 1930's fought with false anecdotal evidence to sell Congress the idea that homicidal mania is linked to Marihuana ingestion.

Pfizer Pharmaceuticals produced a movie, Reefer Madness, likely based on the same tragic event in Ybor City in Tampa Florida. Just as Anslinger used the Ybor City Licata Family Massacre to ramrod his lies so did the movie portrayal of same. Pfizer's movie is one of a genre of twelve films released to the general movie going public in the early part of the nineteen thirties' decade. It showed people going homicidal after smoking Marihuana. Pfizer was putting Bayer aspirin on the market and saw fit to dampen down the competition. One could buy Cannabis in pharmacies from bulk for years and years not counting the five thousand years of positive humon application of both non-psycho active and psycho active Hemp, historically recorded.

Here we are late 2012. The Feds are in California dismantling a few of the state legal Pot growers and dispensaries saying they are selling to non prescription Pot consumers.

Fifteen, make that seventeen now, no eighteen states, TWENTY! and the District of Columbia have passed Medical Marihuana laws. Yet no where, not even Holland, has one hundred percent legal Marihuana. The United States has a long standing treaty with many nations asking them to comply with keeping Pot illegal in return for financial help from the United States. It's called being Pro American.

Bad law doesn't mess around.

It never was a War on Drugs. It has always been a War on People.

1.2.3.4.1.2.3.4.1.2.3.4.1.2.3.4.1.2.3.4.1

The late sixties and the seventies gave us the banner of Sex, Drugs, and Rock 'n Roll. The Baby Boomers were still under twenty five years old. Our young men are being drafted and sent to Vietnam. Peace and Love were fighting for center stage and the powers that be are sending our best and brightest young men off to distant dangerous war. Baby Boomers were and are a massive number of births lasting twelve to eighteen {Depending on the source} years of births. The many births made a population bubble of Americans conceived or born in 1946 and on. Babies made in a country whose Greatest Generation is freshly home from World War II.

To see the Baby Boomer effect picture a skinny snake six feet long as the usual stream of American population numbers. Put a huge Beach Ball inside the snake about two thirds through. The Beach Ball could look a little misshapen as silhouetted to demonstrate weariness at being in the snake for two thirds through, metaphysically speaking.

Post World War II wemun were to be in the home if not barefoot and pregnant at least pregnant as the best way to restore the man as the bread winner in his family. The WASP, White Anglo Saxon Protestant concept of biblical male dominance took the helm. Father got the job of knowing best and wemun used feminine wiles to get their way. This made wemun into successful behind the scene schemers, an unflattering stereotype, unless you love the Lucile Ball incarnation of the 'little womon' on your TV screen. Best fem-ale accolade: Be a 'little womon' toiling away behind your successful man, because behind every successful man is one.

By the early seventies Pot is everywhere. Hair, the musical stage play is making history in New York City.

Hippies are both rich and not rich. Peace and Love are taking hold. Could this be the dawning of The Age of Aquarius? The title of a great popular song about just that. Or, who did not toss away their own internal "Fear of Flying", a ground breaking book title of the era.

The truth is obvious. Pot is harmless, a victimless crime. Pot is beneficial.

The worst thing summoned against it? Cannabis masks symptoms. You'll be feeling fine and unaware of some insidious disease going unattended. More likely you could sail by that insidious disease and remain healthy. No masking, indeed perhaps experiencing more awareness of one's body.

Nay Sayers are persuaded to say Pot is addictive. A substance addiction by definition is physiological. The downside of an addiction is notably due to adverse effects when over consumed or upon attempting abandoning use. Think alcohol, nicotine, caffeine, opiates. Full of toxins to be accommodated by the body. Once accommodated the addiction is on.

Pot, no toxins, is unlawful in public so people who may thrive on Pot are pressured to drop it or never imbibe. Pot's a great choice to imbibe.

To be clear, denying us legal Pot is a Humon Rights Abuse en masse.

No tally of harm to children grown up around Cannabis exists. Not beyond the normal incidences reference non Cannabis families and likely substantially ahead of the alcohol and tobacco using households.

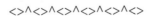

Addiction; the fact or condition of being addicted to a particular substance, thing, or activity.

Addicted; physically and mentally dependent on a particular substance, and unable to stop taking it without adverse effects.

Physiologically; relating to bodily function.

Psychological; of, affecting, or arising in the mind; related to the mental and emotional state of a person; having a mental rather than a physical cause.

Cannabis is not physically addictive. No adverse physical effects known as withdrawal. One may prefer Cannabis imbibing to the point of habituation, no problem, no drug escalation, no hallucinations, no downside beyond the irrational criminalization. Cannabis is a preference. Ask the good people of Washington State and Colorado. No Cannabis related illness(s) exist.

Instead, a long list of attributes for Cannabis grows.

October 18th, 2013, a Washington State Seattle resident interpreted the planned legal twenty one dispensaries selling Pot to replace the current two hundred dispensaries as a big asset for underground sales. Washington State voters legalized recreational Pot in the November 2012 elections.

Psychological addiction arises from a mental or emotional connection that may be worth severing for an individual. Perhaps to pass a pee test? Some few may require outside help to do so. If you are one of those few, get help for the problem. It is a good idea to get help when we can't do something on our own that wants doing.

To demonize Pot, Cannabis, Marijuana/Marihuana, Weed, Grass, or Ganja, by any name, requires a foray into lies and duplicity.

THC, the active ingredient in Cannabis, does not pass into a fetus in the womb through the placenta. An unborn child gets no effect. Nor has second hand Pot smoke proven deleterious. Children grow up unharmed.

Language manipulation and distorted facts are the substance behind the persecution of Cannabis people. Not without standing is the unconstitutional yet enacted criminalizing of non criminals. <u>Shame on all of us for such Congressional ignorance going unaddressed</u>. A legal criminalization of otherwise innocent Americans requires an Amendment to our very Constitution. Two thirds of two thirds of our state level legislators must vote for an Amendment for it to become law. That and only that constitutes a legal Prohibition that criminalizes people.

As it is we toil for Efficacy Proof for Medicinal Marijuana of some caliber beyond the obvious. It's needed as soon as possible. The proof must appear as an accredited scientific study that finds Marijuana Medicinal, a blessing. Let it be forthwith and forthcoming and read with approval by a decider at the DEA, the Federal Government Drug Enforcement Agency.

&*&*&*&*&*&*&*&*&*&*&*&*&

Peace. Let's choose Peace.

Potheads know Cannabis for the health restorative it is.

The sex, drugs and rock 'n roll Boomers became the center of attention by virtue of their massive numbers and by being the focus of merchandisers everywhere. Boomer influence appeared to be taking shape in spite of the dreadful overseas Vietnam War lasting years and years set to demoralize and devastate Boomer political cohesiveness. We witnessed over a decade of the munching up of our young men sent to war. Again the need to squash Boomer influence on the culture becomes paramount because Boomers are aging into becoming politically cohesive.

If you tune into Fox News television regularly you are unlikely to be reading this page. Distortion and fear pushed by hyper emotional presentation meant to inflame rather than inform viewers. . . Pathetic.

Back in the sixties and early seventies the norm soon morphed from peace and love to duck and cover on the home front, most especially if you were non white. The Boomers became a big threat to the status quo. Big War, and therefore Big Oil, Big Pharmaceuticals, Big Government, the powers that be, got the message: divide and conquer, decimate the cohesion of the young Boomers.

The culture itself had a terrific solution, turn Hippies into Yuppies. Hippies in tie-died clothing were doing communes and food coops and anti-war movements, and loved Pot. Many Hippies turned in their tie-dye for a coat and tie, male and female, witness the movie Annie Hall. Yuppies went straight. They wore real shoes, marking the return of wingtips, and turned in their educations for executive salaries and "keeping up with the Jones", an old expression for conspicuous consumption. We know this phenomenon as two cars in every driveway and within a decade the seventies launched the two income family required by the eighties, to keep pace.

The Vietnam War surviving participants came home bent and broken to suffer again at the culture's hands. Sixty five thousand Vietnam soldiers, mostly Boomers, died in Vietnam. Boomer ex-soldiers were as damaged then as the ex-soldiers from our two wars this century, Iraq and Afghanistan, only without the sympathy. No cohesiveness of Boomers, Hippies, or Peace and Love influence survived into the eighties.

HIV, also known as AIDS, took out freely enjoyed sex. 'Drugs' got you arrested or unemployed. Rock n Roll lives on.

$%$%$%$%$%$%$%$

All 'drugs' are bad. How we all managed to accept the word 'drugs' as horrific when we buy drugs at a drug store is a masterpiece of Public Relations, don't you think?

In the Tampa Tribune newspaper August 18th, 2013 in a commentary written by Paul Guzzo we learn an astonishing Truth. The core or the legislation against Cannabis dates to a specific misappropriated tragic event whose perpetrator was a known severely mentally ill individual whose evil rampage of hacking a family of innocent people to death in their home became a ramrod for Pot criminalization.

One Henry Anslinger, then head of the Federal Bureau of Narcotics took this tragic event in October 1933 in Tampa's Ybor City to be his banner of cause for including Marihuana in the United States Congressional Narcotics Tax Act of 1937. The Licata Family's Killer was said to have killed because of Pot use. Anslinger provided two hundred negative Pot related anecdotal stories, the ax killing of the Licata Family on the masthead.

Anslinger brought to his crusade two hundred examples of people wild and evil on Marihuana. Each one failed to check out and is debunked as invalid, we're told.

"It may never be known why he, [Anslinger] lied, but there is no denying he did." as written by Paul Guzzo in the Tampa Tribune story retold in print, August 2013.

Why did Anslinger lie? One popular theory holds his motivation was to benefit the DuPont family industry making petroleum oil based house paint. Dupont industries led the fiber and paper Industrialists, who were at the time looking at upcoming active competition from Hemp's growing popularity with Dupont's competition, other fiber based product manufacturers. The DuPonts are Anslinger's friends.

The Tampa Tribune story of the Licata Family massacre sheds light on the lynchpin of Marihuana demonization.

This is ground breaking information. It's proven. There is no basis for the initial legislation that criminalized Marihuana. The crime is punishing us with an invalid law. No subsequent bad outcomes impugn Pot. Obviously ruining lives by making an asset to the humon condition outlawed must cease and desist forthwith.

We are counting on you, Eric Holder, Attorney General.

We expect freedom to be instituted during your administration, President Obama, sir.

Consider one could point to the ten thousand newly dead every year victims from drunk drivers for anecdotal evidence for criminalization of alcohol. But that Prohibition failed us miserably, didn't it?

The Federal Drug Enforcement Agency kept reclassification of Pot at bay yet again in January 2013. Cannabis is a Schedule I Drug. Right there with the opiates and resultant Felony sentencing, the worst. Nothing considered beneficial or medicinal allowed.

An appeals court voted two to one to agree with the Drug Enforcement Agency assertion that any proof of the efficacy of Marihuana as medicinally beneficial is non-existent. Imagine, non-existent, the DEA said. No efficacy proof as a medicinal substance. Did they look in all their DEA file cabinets?

So we are forced to procure Pot illegally, some of us locked up for years over the mere uningested presence of an innocent vegetation with provable efficacy.

There is no proof in our known reality existing that Pot turns good people into criminals. How on God's Green Earth can the lack of being proven to the DEA's satisfaction, Marihuana's medicinal efficacy, is adequate as the backbone for the DEA's persistence arresting American citizens to the tune of one million plus annually, is incomprehensible Hog Wash!

Efficacy or no efficacy, why make people into felons over Pot? Pot is an Historically Proven, Creation Given, Natural Resource, Health Restorative, Superior Libation and Environmental Asset.

Non-existent DEA, more like.

Note: Canada allows growing non psycho active Hemp, America does not. Americans may not grow even non psycho active Hemp to this day. Canada does a brisk business growing Hemp for industry. England produces vastly superior building blocks for homes using Hemp. See later in this book more remarks about a new product called Hemp Crete. Hemp Crete is used to build homes far superior for insulation and fire protection. Known superior especially for being so non allergenic. It's prohibitively expensive for Americans to use Hemp Crete to build a home because Hemp Crete is produced in England. One Hemp Crete home is in Florida so far, we've heard.

Consider the Narcotics Tax Act of 1937 effectively shut down scientific inquiry into the properties of Pot in this country. Permits are required to do a legitimate study and very few have been allowed over the decades. Yes, we now know Marihuana has no toxins. No intoxication, no shutting down from poison as from alcohol, no inherent carcinogenic components. We know Marihuana is far from dangerous compared to nicotine and legal prescription drugs. Prescription drugs of any ilk are not clean of toxins. There will be negative side effects for every laboratory made drug consumed, be it a pronounced side effect or miniscule.

Nowadays one may purchase synthetic Pot over the counter. K-2 it's called. It appears to be much more powerful and may actually be addictive physically, unlike the real Cannabis plant consumed. K-2 has a patent and money is being made.

An update could prove additional legislation is in place against synthetic Pot.

There is no legal handling of Marihuana. It's contraband. A criminalized beneficial vegetation. Clear injustice, a Humon* Rights Violation amounting to Persecution, for which there is no defense. Current demonization of Cannabis is merely empty words painting frightening hypothetical unforeseeable outcomes. Words said and pictures painted for one result, to prevent inclusion when liberty and justice for all, and scientifically proven truth, prove inclusion is wisdom. Be reminded, inclusion IS our directive for survival: personal, the masses, and the planet's.

olioliolioliolioliolioliolo

Taxpayers are paying for political prisoners to be caught and kept in jails in order to keep the Underworld, Big Pharmaceuticals, Big Oil and the rest, all happy with the status quo of not questioning the BIG LIE of Cannabis as dangerous.

We keep Big Government and Big Business Happy, too. All the while we are making prisoners out of non criminal individuals over a denied beneficial substance. This is unjust and reprehensible. Individuals, American citizens, suffer needlessly. Ludicrous. At the expense of the ninety nine percent 1.6 million Americans were arrested on Marihuana charges in 2010. Over a Million Americans arrested both 2011 and 2012.

Pot's nemesis spokes people are reduced to saying the danger of Pot legalization resides with the adolescent user purported to drop I.Q. points from Cannabis consuming.

If there is only the one study ever mentioned to support this loose remark at best, it is the one with a mere forty people divided heavy Pot consumers versus non Pot users. A measure of their brain's dopamine, a brain chemical neurotransmitter, showed less dopamine in the Pot users brains. The negative extrapolation of the results stated a eight point I.Q. drop for adolescents who consumed Pot. THC, considered Pot's active ingredient, likely substitutes nicely for dopamine as an anticipated brain chemical due to our brains having receptors for THC built in. Won't sell much lab produced Epinephrine with that truth proven.

Dopamine is the precursor for Epinephrine, an adrenaline synthetic that constricts blood vessels and opens airways.

Pot, contraband, whose attributes could conceivably free us from the narrow perception of the current health care model to embracing a Creation Given Natural Resource Health Restorative. Hmmm? Marihuana might relieve us of so much minor, the usually not deadly, health issues like headaches and arthritis to the point of cure.

We will take the chance of legal Pot consumption to see behind the curtain, as in OZ. We know and love the truth here in America where we Pledge Allegiance to Liberty and Justice for all.

*Please note the improved spelling of the word human to humon, as inclusive, singular anyone in general or in particular. This is necessary for our children to no longer need to infer the fem-ale gender as included and lesser.

Womon for woman
Wemun for Women
Man, when only one man
Men, if only males
Monkind = Mankind
Humonity = Humanity
Humon = Human
Humuns = Humans
Humone = Humane
Humunity = Humanity

Mon: new word meaning an anonymous man or a
    womon singular,
    Example:
    "It's every Mon for himself."
Mun: new word meaning anonymous men and womun,
    all of us, grouped or not
    Example:
    "All good Mun must come to the aid of the Party."

Amun = Amen
Fem-ale = female

Evolution of our language is always with us. Language informs us to our very soul. Changing the spelling as above corrects an imbalance of power at a fundamental level. Children steeped in intrinsic gender equality will have mutual respect and build less combative lives together perhaps.

###############

Suppose you find yourself the subject of a Pot bust. While submitting completely to the arrest procedure you say "You are unlawfully intruding into my life based on a False Premise. I know my rights. Therefore I am also making an arrest. I arrest you, {the law enforcement officer(s), now alleged perpetrator(s)} for this unlawful intrusion into my life without Just Cause. I am not a criminal, I am a lifetime non criminal. [say only when so] Marihuana is a Creation Given, Natural Resource, Health Restorative."

"You have the right to remain silent. Anything you say may be used against you in a court of law. You have the right to legal representation. If you cannot afford a lawyer the court will provide a court appointed lawyer for you. Do you understand?" That's the Miranda Rights statement, a must for a legal arrest.

Ask for or work to get the names and badge numbers of the law enforcement alleged perpetrators and follow through with the citizen's arrest procedures as far as possible. One individual to imitate is the immortalized Rosa Parks. She plays a staring role in kick starting a major societal change. Maybe it will take a volume of attempted citizen arrests of law enforcement perpetrators. Pot will soon be riding on the bus, a legitimate choice for health restoration and maintenance, relaxing or energizing.

There is no basis in our law for persecuting individuals whose so called crime relates to providing by cultivating, buying, selling, or possessing a vegetation with no toxic implications or criminal behavior results. The Local, State and Federal Governments must be made to attempt to defend this un-American practice of falsely maintaining the public is served by protecting them from legally obtained Pot. There is no case to be made, no acceptable defense. In twenty states doctors are prescribing Pot to people who are not subsequently crashing their cars, stealing from their employers, abusing their families more than non Potheads. There is no behavior criminally affecting others in any way that demands the removal of Pot or Potheads from normal everyday life as a public service.

Pot is good for people, good for the people who choose to eat or inhale good Weed. It will never be proven otherwise.

Our very brains come equipped with THC receptors!!! It's science. Pot is the key in the lock. Maybe THE key to that dormant ninety percent of our brain power we don't access. There are reams of anecdotal and scientific proof of Pot's medicinal benefits.

None in the hands of the DEA, apparently. This must be remedied.

Criminalization of people in the immediate vicinity of Cannabis is one hundred percent Humon Rights Abuse. Criminalization nets exorbitant tax free Dollars for the contraband marketers and entrenches massive corruption besides hurting and killing those caught in the actual crossfire. The failed efforts of law enforcement to stem the growth of contraband sales, but instead to largely be the cause of the growth, is all at the American taxpayer's expense.

There is a better way.

Remember who we are. We are the people who Pledge our Allegiance to the Flag of the United States of America and to the Country for which it stands, One Nation, Under God, with LIBERTY AND JUSTICE FOR ALL.

Digression:

February 25th, 2012: the current fuss over Florida's Governor Rick Scott's plan to urine test for contraband all Florida State employees has become a, to be legislated, required ten percent of the state employee workforce to undergo random computer generated choosing of individuals to provide a urine sample for a test searching for contraband. Picture the surprise if a top producing employee has to be given the boot over a positive result. Or will the random employees be given some time before the test to avail themselves of the products that cleanse urine of contra banded Cannabis?

All that's needed to agree this unwarranted invasion of an American citizen's privacy is a plus for the good of the state's taxpaying public is for the Governor of Florida to bring forward the proof that the public is being harmed by the previously unknown randomly discoverable contraband in state employee urine, not known up to now.

The bill failed in the courts by fall. . . The promoters of the bill continue trying.

OPEN LETTER TO PRESIDENT
BARRACK OBAMA, 7.20.12

Dear Mr. President,

An opportunity is uniquely yours. You may pardon all the incarcerated, paroled, on probation, every single individual presently or formally charged with a strictly

Cannabis so called offense. Pardon the growers, traffickers, sellers, buyers and possessors, all the people with an offense based on Cannabis. Free Cannabis for all our use. Begin the era of Truth, Equal Rights and Justice. Worldwide.

The nasty repercussions of continuing the systematic demonizing and criminalization of this Creation Given Natural Resource Health Restorative and Superior Libation can end. The lie that Cannabis is not an asset to the humon condition is over.

The perpetuation of the lie is such an enormous force that once reckoned with and set aside it will be as though the kingpin of oppression, manipulation and greed is brought down. Done properly, downing this kingpin will take out the entire set of pins eliminating organized crime from a place of tyranny. Plus, potentially inadvertently solving our health care financial crisis by increasing the health quotient of our people is worth all manner of senseless flack.

Everybody knows the truth. It is not hidden. Cannabis helps people, it does not damage people.

It comes to you, President Obama, please, to choose to be the instrument of change. Correct the falsehood. Admit that America, a shinning star of western civilization and democracy, leader of the free world, has erred. It is time to admit our shame and take back all our demands to other countries to also criminalize Cannabis.

This law, policy, treaty condition and inane derailment of truth and justice goes out with the trash.

Pardon all as stated then ask the people and leaders of all the world to forgive us for our misguided dastardly ways vies a vi Cannabis also known as Marijuana or Pot.

It's a good job done. -MKH

Well, Presidential pardons are subject to review by Congress. Apparently President Obama gets one in about two hundred requested pardons approved, nowhere near the average for Presidents over all for closer to one in thirty. . . . sigh.

One may notice the word humon, aka human, is an inclusive word for men and wemun, visually and to the ear. An overdue improvement. Let's make the change, our children may not thank us, but gender inclusiveness will grow our children immersed in the equality of the sexes.

QQQQQQQQQQQQQQQQQQQQQQQQQQ

October 20, 2012, NPR, National Public Radio had a guest mention that the top one percent of Americans currently make three hundred fifty thousand dollars plus, taxable annual income, as an individual or qualifies as in the top one percent with assets of seven million dollars or more.

rprprprprprprprprprprprpr

Let Law Enforcement accountability begin. How is it valuable to literally hound out of the many the individuals who prefer a creation given natural resource health restorative and superior libation, psycho active Hemp?

So much office space and paid for work relates to and surrounds tracking and capturing defendants in The Drug War, as it's known to lay people.

To the law makers it's a Title: The Drug Abuse Prevention and Control Act-1970, under the Food and Drugs Title 21, USC Chapter 13, -EXPCITE-, 01/03/2012, or as updated.

This whole aspect of discussion is covered by the Severability Paragraph set into Subchapter I, page ten of a two hundred seventy page printout of The Drug Abuse Prevention and Control Act-1970. President Nixon is in the Whitehouse.

Here, again, is the whole enchilada: Quote of a printed "quote" under Severability, it reads:

Severability

Quote entered as law: 114 Stat. 1246, provided that: "Any provision of this title {see Short Title Of 200 Amendments note above} held to be invalid or unenforceable by its terms, or as applied to any person or circumstance, shall be constructed as to give the maximum effect permitted by law, unless such provision is held to be utterly invalid or unenforceable, in which event such provision shall be severed from this title, and shall not affect the applicability of the remainder of this title, or of such provision, to other persons not similarly situated or to other, dissimilar circumstances."

October 17, 2000, Pub. L. 106-310, div. B, title XXXVI, Sec. 3673.

Nothing else, period the end. On to the next, easy pezy. Hmmmmm.

INVALID [Bad Law and Policy] and UNENFORCEABLE [Innocent People Persecuted]? Okay, sever the bad law and policy because it targets the innocent, only this changes, it's gone. Drop The Cannabis Prohibition. 1,2,3, A,B,C, Abracadabra, ipso facto, Please and Thank you, GONE!

De Facto! No more illegality, just like tomatoes and catsup, is Pot. Your family will find and choose it's own path. With or without Cannabis.

That's the whole enchilada: Employ Severability, the legal escape clause, literally, for Marihuana to leave criminalization behind.

eferusroferusroferusroferusroferusrofe

The US Schedule I Drug Cannabis: in a more than a Misdemeanor amount, usually fifteen or more grams, Caught? Felony Charge. An ounce is twenty eight grams. If arrested fifteen grams is a prosecutable Felony, a serious criminal offense. Three strikes of the mandatory three felony strikes and you are jailed for life without parole, very serious.

FELONY: a crime, typically one involving violence, regarded as more serious than a misdemeanor, and usually punishable by imprisonment for more than one year or by death.

MISDEMEANOR: a minor wrongdoing. In Law, a non indictable offense.

INDICTABLE: (of an offense) rendering the person who commits it liable to be charged with a serious charge that warrants a trial by jury, (of a person). Liable to be charged with a crime.

Then there is Drug Court, likely unconstitutional. The establishing of a court along side the Judicial Branch of Government is outside our rule of law as written which forbids any such establishment thus making Drug Court untenable. One immediately recognizes that if you want to punish someone it has to be a crime according to written established law containing the legal protections as provided, so the accused remains innocent until proven guilty by peers forming a jury in a traditional court of law, with a revealed accuser. Defense presented.

Once we bring back justice there will be no Drug Court, where no exonerating defense is allowed. No one leaves unscathed.

It makes unsubstantiated as criminal perpetrators, the humon fodder, called clients, as each is marched through the drug court, a victim of perhaps unconstitutional procedures. Drug Court Judges decree jail time, probations and counseling, rehab, community service. Often all the aforementioned.

The Probationers are required to pass a urine test to avoid being hauled off to jail immediately at the point of a failed urine test at the Corrections Department where each reports when on probation. Probationers are tested each visit. Fail your pee test? Yes, the hand cuffs go on. The individual formerly on probation goes directly to jail in the cage style back seat of a Police Car to serve a sentence, to again come out on probation, to again fail a pee test to again go back to jail in minutes from failing the pee test.

Yes, there are uncontrolled controlled substances in prisons. All this tax payer paid humon abuse is based on the individual's positive test result showing urine tainted with THC. Or perhaps it's tainted with another contraband. Probationers are tested every time they see a probation officer at the local Corrections Department where the convicted must frequently report as well as opening their homes for drop by visits. Probationers receive an additional prison sentence for not staying clean for a urine test.

Besides probations, detainees are offered plea bargaining to bring their sentence down to a probation. The men get reduced sentences more often than the busted wemun because the men have names to give up for additional busts where as the wemun are not privy to having an informant's knowledge, thus the wemun with little or no involvement get longer sentences than the men from the same bust.

Being in the judicial penal system, as a convicted felon means a total lost of privacy in the convicted person's home and life. Felons remain persons of interest forever, the first to be matched to any other crime in the search for a perpetrator.

So much persecution, all based on an indefensible falsely premised contra banding of so called controlled substances.

At the very least it is easy to see that the twenty eight million Americans plus who enjoy Marihuana and all the vendors, growers and traffickers who are state legal are showing us the absurdity of the sincerely felonious activity of law enforcement attempting to rid America of Cannabis consumers, supremely innocent people as far as the Cannabis consumption goes. Never been otherwise.

254&*$*$3214676qq69

Congratulations to Reelected President Barrack Obama. Congratulations to the people of Washington and Colorado for legalizing Marihuana for recreational use. The people of Colorado endorsed legalization in part because they expect the state to collect big tax dollars. Now begins the process of sorting out the details. Consider the legal ounce an individual may now possess in these two states since the new law's passage. Only Federal law still criminalizes the Grower, Trafficker and Seller. Tax belongs at the point of sale. More unfolding history in the saga that is our march to a civil society.

Clarity. Late August 2013 President Obama tells federal prosecutors of Pot possessions to reflect the legalization of Pot per the State in question. The People's Rights as legislated legalizing Pot are to be instituted and therefore shall no longer be of concern to the federal government for prosecution.

############

The white people of the world took a hit on their long standing superiority when the United States Constitution no longer said blacks are only four fifths humon. Hit again as Hitler's ilk lost World War II. Another hit came as the ex-one term governor of Massachusetts, Mitt Romney lost his bid for Presidency of the United States in November 2012 to incumbent President Barrack Obama, a so called black man as his father is a native African from Kenya, college educated state side, thus fathering Barrack Obama with his Kansas born wife, a white person.

The vote tabulation done demographically revealed Mitt's overwhelmingly white constituency.

The hit coming next? Marihuana acceptance by the government.

Perhaps Marihuana is legalized de facto now.

De facto in hopes of nipping in the bud the following: A Pot head steps out, camps in a Florida State Park. A monned Sniffer Dog detects THC, any narcotic, on a camper bath house visitor. The dog tracts same to the burnt Cannabis scented camper's camp site.

The Sniffer Dog sits down, the alert.

A quantity of law enforcement arrive. Who knows how many. The assailed tax paying law abiding citizen does expose the tiny stash of Pot and the pipe used on site in their tent on the rented for two nights land.

The assailed individual responds thusly to the words of an arrest. Apparently the camper's leaving the park, no further harassment by the law, is not to be considered sufficient.

The camper's response:

"Officer(s), I in no way resist your arrest. I do also place you under Citizen's Arrest for intruding into my life and my inalienable right to Life, Liberty and the pursuit of Happiness. Officer(s), you are acting on a False Premise. Pot is not by definition and practice a Class A Schedule I Drug as defined by the United States Federal government.

Miranda rights spoken by Camper here: "Dear Officer(s), having relieved me of my Liberty I place you under Citizen Arrest. Prove your Just Cause to relieve me of my Liberty.

You have the right to remain silent. Anything you say can and will be used against you in a court of law. You are entitled to legal representation. You may have a court appointed lawyer if unable to provide your own legal representation."

The governments, local, state or federal, any arresting officer represents as taxpayer supported and funded law enforcement may not proceed arresting innocent American citizens without first proving Cannabis as possessed is a substance with no positive applications for humon health and no known medicinal attributes as proven by the voting public and medical doctor endorsement. We know from repeated public endorsement, the people or state legislators of state after state, twenty times over, by fall 2013 endorse Pot itself and even recreational users in two states. The public is voting for and has enjoyed for years and years Pot use that only a blatant hypocrite or bigot or person paid to persecute would revile.

You may not legally harm a Preamble and Constitutionally protected Pothead for being a Pothead any more legitimately than keeping people sitting close to the rear of public buses by reason of skin color.-MKH

Potheads belong to be allowed on the "legitimate" bus openly. There is no case against Pot or Potheads.

False Premise: Pot is a legitimate Class A Schedule I Drug.

Pot deserves to flow as freely as tomatoes in the marketplace. Regulate commercial taxable sales.

The legitimacy of truth is integral to the American Way.

Defense of persecution is groundless. This entire treatise is to equip the reader to speak up and knowledgeably answer back the ignorant and uninformed. Even as the obvious emerges, momentum is necessary to gain legitimacy status.

Pot is best known as an asset to the humon condition.

&&&&&&&&&&&&&&&&&&&&&&&

White people are losing the biggest hammer of oppression, illegal Cannabis. Criminalization of a beneficial Herb makes a tool for clouting us down into a well controlled beaten down and not rich populace, fertile cheap labor. Non white American numbers already are a majority and are growing.

Relax white people. As long as you are willing to observe all of us as equal and deserving of respect, you will be respected and deserving of equality.

That's the Beauty of Truth and Justice. Eventually Truth and Justice Triumph and everyone Wins. This is the American Way.

OKOKOKOKOKOKOKOKOKOKOKOKO

November 26th, 2012, The United States Supreme Court, the highest court in our land, is hearing a case to decide if a home dweller has a right to our Constitution's 4th Amendment protections from intrusion, in particular from a narcotics sniffing Police dog search without a warrant.

Does an uninvited policeperson with a narcotic sniffing dog coming to one's front door, constitute probable cause to search, if the dog alerts?

This up from a Florida Case pertaining to a dog's "alert" due to possible contraband in a vehicle that revealed something not in that dog's trained repertoire. The Florida Supreme Court ruled this dog to be improperly credentialed, so the case is found for the defendant. Now the case is brought to the United States Supreme Court because law enforcement wants to pursue contraband possession with narcotic sniffing dogs everywhere, including any front porch.

What are the attributes of keeping Pot contraband? Why does no one on the high court question the validity of persecuting individuals for Pot possession when the will of the people to legally use Marihuana builds momentum visibly?

Who knows one example of a general malaise of any sort that defines the criminality of Pot possession and use?

In fact the individuals who are affected by the consequence of this ruling to come ought to be considered.

The law enforcement speakers in that Florida Courtroom as they presented their case, had nothing to say about the alleged perpetrators to be handcuffed and removed without further liberty supposedly to be charged with a crime eligible for jail time. For an alleged perpetrator many scenarios may ensue.

The quality and duration of the unfolding events of an arrest are dependent on the defendant's wealth and luck or lack thereof.

Most of the would be defendants, now Drug Court Clients, will be fodder in a, likely unconstitutional Drug Court. There is little chance of incarceration for a first offense misdemeanor conviction on up to plea bargaining to reduce a possible horrendous jail time sentence for a felony charge. One snitches on others for reduced sentencing.

One Supreme Court Justice mentioned the harm done when a dog alerts on a vehicle with no contraband in evidence when searched. It sounded like a good Sniffer Dog is considered reliable at seventy percent correct or a near F failing grade in humon terms. One opinion heard stated searched houses, cars and people, searched erroneously for narcotics, can turn up other offenses, thus making for police work. Law enforcement opines searching itself is worthwhile because of the found offenses. No home content privacy for citizens in that opinion.

The Supreme Court has long since ruled that the FBI, the Federal Bureau of Investigation, may enter an American individual's home surreptitiously without the home dweller's knowledge, in the course of conducting a fact finding investigation. Legally. Be the homeowner sound asleep or not home.

The Supreme Court could rule for the same appropriateness of surreptitious searches for any law enforcement investigation just to speed things up and avoid wasting time and money. Hypothetically.

We grapple world wide with the NSA, National Security Agency, as it prowls thru all of everybody's digital communication data, mega data gathering with sifting programs in place. Chancellor Markel of Germany is miffed over her loss of privacy on her phone.

Surreptitious searches, Phooey. But think how efficient a police state could be and we are already so close to our government in total becoming a totalitarian system. Even now an individual's stake on truth and justice is hanging by a thread.

Witness the Supreme Court ruling to make virtually unlimited in the name of free speech the amount of money a contributor may give a candidate. From one hundred twenty six thousand over a two year election cycle to two million dollars per person, infinite candidates. No more frustrated billionaires. April 2,2014.

Signs of we the people rousing ourselves for a pull on our government to taking care of important matters such as decent laws: A PEW Service Poll significant enough for National Public Radio to make it news reports sixty seven percent of all polled favor legalizing drugs, Schedule I drugs. Legalizing the hard drugs and Marijuana both, favored. Only twenty six percent were against any legalization. This poll covered enough demographics to make it a serious take on public sentiment it was said. April 2, 2014.

One radio NPR reporter concluded while a third of us may still see the drug scourge as a crisis even they don't think prison is the answer.

Update: The NSA, National Security Agency, has an errant leaker, Edward Snowden, now ensconced in Russia. The latest revealed intrusion into our privacy came early

September, 2013. We find out the most thought to be securely protected for privacy, electronic personal info, of people and businesses, has been hacked by a tax supported government entity. Aggravating to many. When it comes to prying and spying The NSA knows no bounds. Congress is playing caught unaware, too. Yet the United States Congressional Patriot Act of 2004 created the NSA to have access to 'any tangible thing', then Congress added anytime and carte blanche funding for all the spying.

0!0!0!0!0!0!0!0!0!0!0!0

As long as the federal government fails to demonstrate to the American people any as yet unknown gain made for the American public by contra banding Pot, or any other verboten bit of nature, we are living a lie.

Making criminals out of Marihuana possessors is nothing more than the crime of persecution. We Americans deserve and now must demand better treatment of our people. Remember, our constitution guarantees the right of anyone to stake out their own parameters as long as they don't harm another.

If we used a harm index to attempt to eliminate the most obvious damagers to the consuming public and the public at large, alcohol and tobacco would be illegal, instantly.

Meanwhile Pot has great credentials. Better to close the Gate, separate the hard drugs from the medicinal and recreational Marihuana. As it is we are denied an obvious asset to the humon condition and the endless contraband sellers have entry to people of all ages everywhere no regulation, carte blanche lawlessness and big tax free profits. Surely the recognition of what and who is wrong is revealed.

Heroin has come back to gain huge ground in the last two years, sad to say. It's said cocaine users are converted to heroin by their cocaine dealers.

.%K%.%K%.%K%.%K%.%K%.%K%.

December 6, 2012, Marihuana is mainstream news. The day begins the first day the people of Washington state may smoke in private legally. The Feds intervention in the purchase process once the state's licensing of growers and vendors and tax income flows, seems moot. Potheads may get Driving Under the Influence apprehensions, likely ending in arrests, if their blood tests positive for THC, the active ingredient in Cannabis. THC content exceeding five milligrams per five milliliters of blood is the expressed excessive amount.

End of August 2013, President Obama spoke to us of the change in the Directive to Federal Prosecutors in the legalized Pot states. He said the people in those states will not be raided or charged in accordance with their state laws over Cannabis. Not all prosecutors are prepared to change.

The Washington State Police have weighted in saying they will stop a driver driving badly. They won't be seeking out Potheads.

In Florida a white haired senior citizen fellow, Robert Platshorn, is traveling the state touting the attributes of Marihuana as remedy for the ailments of aging. The Daily Show with Jon Stewart showed an interview by Al Madrigal.

The show aired Wednesday, December 6, 2012. The televised clips show Robert Platshorn lecturing rows of seniors who finished the event munching Pot laced foods provided by the host. Here's a list provided by Mr. Platshorn of twenty medical Marihuana uses:

Huntington's Disease
ALS
HIV
Alzheimer's Disease
Dystonia
Sleep Apnea
MSRE
Fibromyalgia
Hepatitis C
Osteoporosis
Rheumatoid Arthritis
GI Disorders
Gliomas/Cancer
Chronic Pain
Incontinence
Diabetes Mellitus
Purities
Torrents Syndrome
Hypertension
Multiple Sclerosis

<M><M><M>M><M><M><M?><M><M><M><M>

On an historical note, there was a determined prejudice against tea consumption in parts of the British Isles going back hundreds of years that still has remnants in evidence in the Irish Isles. Tea was said to be the cause of hankering by virtue of it's addictive nature. Black Teas have caffeine naturally. This subject is researched by Helen O'Connell, as interviewed on National Pubic Radio.

Hmm, and many Americans also wish for a tea time every afternoon at four PM, scones and all. Each to their own.

We people of the world can appreciate the passing of nonsense as far as a taboo on tea goes apparently.

The first week of December 2012 shows no relenting of the Non Democratic party, read Tea Party Republicans. They will not accept letting go the tax cuts for the top two percent of all Americans, our wealthy. At this juncture our wobbly barely past the deep Bush Recession economy after the Bush 2008 mortgage debacle and subsequent recession here, the recession in Europe, shrinking growth in China, injustice in the Middle East, all needs a steady hand to steer us to deeper, less hazardous waters, hull in-tack. Real crisis must trump the hypothetical.

Deal with the one real crisis with some cuts, get the usual Tax Revenue from the rich again, spend on infrastructure, all as is laid out in the solution for our budget. Yes, five hundred billion dollars for infrastructure is part of the Obama Administration's solution. We are trying to educate our congressmon to stop dodging their work as legislators hired to make progress, and stop the intolerable routine blackmailing of the public by refusing to face up to established obligations endorsed by the public and do the work in their job descriptions.

Rome wasn't built in a day and the ship, the Queen Elizabeth II, can't spin on a dime. Try either one, dumping on our obligations or spinning the QEII and kill the entire enterprise. No more denying us debt ceiling increases.

Keep in mind stressing an immediate urgency to balancing the budget is possibly as damaging as the blind incurrence of a war. The middle class after the Bush Banking Debacle of 2008, whose result is known here as the Great

Bush Recession, sucked off home owner equity. The stealing of our equity and the subsequent drop in Middle Class well being from a lingering deep recession, are potent miseries, 2010.

October 2013, we are getting over the sixteen day Federal Government Shut Down begun the first of the month.

We have a brief reprieve. The debt ceiling raising vote is set to time out again in January 2014. The Republicans are blamed for the heinous Shut Down costing ten billion dollars a week. Perhaps we will see an improvement in our legislators behavior. We need actual legislation such as immigration law reform, tax loop holes closed, infrastructure and education funded. Fix up the Affordable Health Care Act as is reasonable and anticipated.

Our House of Representatives, by ignoring responsible leadership make us identify with another comedic team. They were paid to be truly entertaining screw-ups.

"This is another <u>fine</u> <u>mess</u> you've [read government, and the lack there of] gotten us into." says Hardy of Laurel & Hardy fame, while characteristically flipping the bottom half of his tie at us watching on the screen. He speaks for us all. October, 2013.

Still haven't heard a ruling from the Supreme Court on the so called Narcotics Sniffer Dogs use on a citizen residence doorstep to establish probable cause for a warranted search if the dog alerts for contra banded drugs. The Supreme Court may take the option not to rule.

Hint: Keep those hands washed. Dogs sniff car door handles and doorknobs in particular.

8888888888888888888888888

North Korea is a great candidate as a test kitchen for an all out diplomatic seduction of it's population. December 12th, 2012, North Korea successfully launched a four stage rocket. Put on a nuclear payload and forget it. Short range?

ooooooooooooooooo

Folks in Colorado celebrate Recreational Pot legalization. They illegally smoked in public without reprisal one day.

An individual said in that moment, "It smells like Freedom."

One ounce is now legal in private in Colorado, especially celebrated one week day, December 11th, 2012. The Public Broadcasting System News Hour Show interviewed a holding company owner of a Growing Facility and a nine product line Production Facility of THC laced Dixie Elixirs, the brand name. Both of those facilities are located in the heart of Denver. All his products are going out as Medical Marihuana, with thirty five million dollars in sales annually. His business is set to morph huge with recreational use legal.

Pot tourism is anticipated in Colorado.

March 18, 2013: The people of Colorado still wait for the roll out of taxation reference their legal Cannabis possession recently passed, no doctor required. Exciting.

Repeated update: President Obama directs States having Pot legalization no longer prosecute Pot per the new state laws legalizing Pot. Federal law is set aside in those twenty states and the District of Columbia, Washington.

The business of Congress is at a standstill, still. Our moribund Congress gave us The Sequestration. It lowers non-defense discretionary spending by a range of 7.8% in 2013 to 5.5% in 2021. This is the food for kids' lunches and educational programs being cut. Check this on Wickipedia. The Sequestration that arbitrarily cuts funding across the board kicked in March 1, 2013.

Receiving Federal Money? Minus money these days unless it's Social Security or Medicaid. Medicare is cut 2% a year for the next eight years. Surprisingly the first weeks of Sequestration cuts sustaining is hardly noticed, except in spotty ways, with momentum gaining. The more obvious crunch is projected as more noticeable summer, 2013. Because Congress is not performing it appears the Sequestration cuts will remain in place to become the norm for the whole eight years.

President Obama is courting Congress to convince them, the Democrats and Republicans in the United States House of Representatives, to work together to do the requisite give and take. They ought to quickly get us past financial-debt-paying-cliff-hanging-budgeting for more than a few weeks. The populace appears to have adjusted. The scariness of the ride into our foreseeable economic future is verging on intense when not going strong for shareholders. The DOW, our usual stock market barometer has bounced a tiny bit over the rigidity of Congress, actually recovering to new heights after the end of the sixteen day mostly Shut Down United States Government. Funding of our government was held hostage by the House of Representatives right up to the brink of a portended Debt Default because of a failure to raise the Debt Ceiling to pay appropriated and committed unpaid expenditures like Treasury Bond interest payments.

Failure to pay our debts is considered by our economically cognizant as a giant step towards doom.

Earlier in 2013 we heard of a big reaction by bank account holders in Europe over a necessary tax being levied on bank accounts on the island of Cypress. They are righting their sinking economic ship. Cypress is a money haven as their main business. So the celebrated new high in the DOW last week flew like a flock of birds with simultaneous liftoff. The cause? The Panicking of those who then created a run on the banks. Thus precipitating the few days of bank closures on Cypress to steady things up.

Currently, we live, eat, drink and be merry with a fragile backdrop of stability because legislators and legislation lack understanding of the worldwide interconnectedness underpinning our mutual survival i.e. our shared successes and untenable failures.

Feed and educate the young, repair the infrastructure and go bravely forth trusting in goodness, dear Congress. Maybe do a little in God We Trust. Hypothetical outcomes tossed aside to bring real solutions to real everyday problem issues. The richest country needs to extinguish hunger before it parades as a leader of the free world. Choose to govern addressing essential priorities for the people. We the people need practical logic not flawed ideology at the helm.

President Obama can deliver if the humons in Congress drop their arrogant ignoramus posturing and get on with spending and investing in a good future for our country that rebuilds the middle class.

Drop the obvious bullying to push the Obama administration into oblivion that is hammering the American people. Good bye Tea Partiers and their main underwriters the Koch brothers. Tank the coup.

vklvklvklvklvklvklvklvklvklvklv

Heard and told as broadcast on NPR, National Public Radio, by a father of a four year old daughter:

"My daughter and I are walking to Central Park. We're on a sidewalk where we pass the steps of each building as we walk. I notice a fella with a doobie he's toking on the steps ahead. As we pass. I say to him, 'I want to 'holler' at you, sir, for a minute.' I take him aside. I say, 'Could you take that (the doobie) somewhere else so when my daughter and I walk by here she doesn't have to smell that?' Of course, he agreed and we parted agreeably."

The 'fella' on the steps smoked a Marihuana joint we are told.

If this father crosses the street to avoid tobacco smoke or covers his daughter's face and ears rather than walk his daughter's exposed orifices that close to a person smoking a tobacco cigarette he will teach his daughter tolerance. Or without avoidance of the tobacco the father risks polluting his baby's ears and/or respiratory system to the point of illness.

The rebuke the father offers to Cannabis is to teach his daughter political correctness while being unwittingly morally reprehensible, enforcing a ban with no just cause.

Defining private property seems easy enough if that is to become the boundary for legal consumption.

We are at a time in history when few know the origin of the demonizing of Cannabis. Marihuana is the name applied to Cannabis for purposes of law in America. Marihuana is Pot in Spanish.

Pfizer Pharmaceuticals sought big sales for Bayer Aspirin. Pfizer Pharmaceuticals took advantage of the popularity of movies in the early 1930's. They, Pfizer, produced the movie Reefer Madness. In this movie a small party of adults in a middle class living room imbibe Cannabis. Soon we see one of the group out in the middle of the street on the way to commit murder. Twelve such movies were made. In 1937, at the last minute, Marihuana was added to the Narcotics Tax Act.

Note this when reading in this book about a Mr. Anslinger. He is the man who got Marihuana criminalized in 1937.

To digress. We are told the thirteen year, legally codified by the 18th Amendment to the United States Constitution, a Total Alcohol Prohibition, bestowed much exaggerated wealth on the illegal providers of booze, making super wealthy criminals.

In turn when the 18th Amendment was repealed in 1933 with the 21st Amendment it took only four years to have a Congress in place bought by Bootlegger Wealth to establish the Narcotics Tax Act of 1937. Thus providing untold wealth and power for those organized criminals pushing opiates evermore.

Accordingly in turn, the persuasive Mr. Anslinger spoke tossing Marihuana into the contraband mix.

Until we wise up. Even now tastes for addictive poison have turned to pharmaceuticals, the laboratory made painkillers. If that is in short supply, cocaine, then heroin. For those who complete the course? A roulette of dosage mishaps.

After the Narcotic Tax Act of 1937 passed, if you are Hispanic, Asian, or Black you are fodder for busting. Got Pot? Proof the Tax was paid? No? Off to jail. And so it went until The Narcotics Tax Act of 1937 received a makeover and became the almost three hundred page book known as the Narcotics Abuse and Prevention Act Of 1970.

Equal Opportunity Pot busts began. Major demonizing of Marihuana took place by linking it to cocaine. Must be bad.

The Feds had had airplanes spray paraquat, a poison dust, on to Pot fields in Mexico. Pot bound for America. Late 1960's.

First Lady, Mrs. Nancy Regan said, "Just Say No".

Thus ushering in America's mid 1980's frontline Drug War. The feebleness of any success managing the zooming addictions to the opiates prohibited by Contraband Schedule I Classified Drugs, ironically including Marihuana, brought gangs across the nation untold wealth, territory defended with bloodshed, including the innocent publics' blood.

Too many people peacefully occupying the inside of their homes lost their lives as innocent 'bystanders'.

Gangs, et.al. answered Mrs. Regan's "Just Say No" campaign with Crack Cocaine mass sales. Same contrary results as the first legal Prohibition on Alcohol. Mammoth escalation of consumption of a dangerous highly addictive drug and mammoth untaxed wealth both took off in earnest.

Thus ended, with a defining coup de grace, legitimate governing. Lies pushed Truth off the table in a media blitz. Marihuana was and is classified as dangerous, called hazardous even, with no known medicinal use. The contrary is soundly proven. As we know, it is medicinal. If danger is the problem adding alcohol and tobacco to Schedule I Drug Classification is level appropriate, as alcohol and tobacco have a hugely greater harm index by number of deaths inflicted than any opiate in the Schedule I Drug Classification.

No Just Cause exists for relieving an individual of their liberty over Cannabis. Not now, not ever.

Cannabis consumers would be joyful to have the rights of tobacco or alcohol consumers. Even caffeine is more harmful than Pot. One can die of a caffeine overdose. No toxins in Cannabis, no deaths, no addiction. Life long preferences to live healthy aided by the THC in Cannabis? Yes.

.8.8.8.8.8.8.8.8.8.8.8.8.8.8.

This book may well contain imperfect numbers and assertions. Your verification is recommended. Google search away. The thrust of this book as intended is to arm anyone who is fed up with the silly manipulation of the public to keep Marijuana contraband. So many states plus the District of Columbia are choosing to legalize Pot if medicinally used and prescribed by a physician and now even recreational use is unfolding in two states. Washington and Colorado legalized recreational Pot by ballot in November 2012, Colorado still waiting for the mechanism for taxation to be in place. How to do this when the Feds supersede with Illegality of Cannabis, still? Hmmmmm. Problem solved, stay tuned.

The District of Columbia passed medical Marihuana three years ago and is now about to be allowed to proceed. Congress had to approve the people's vote. Progress.

Negative headlines are not resulting where people consume state legal medical application Pot. There's no excuse left. Science tells us we are all born with receptors in our brains for THC. Most recently again proven by long distance runners whose bodies make THC. THC is the psycho active component of Cannabis.

Cannabis is a God Given Natural Recourse Health Restorative and Superior Libation, Easily grown and environmentally friendly. It will not be mandatory when legal. Although it is likely to become known as an antidote to tobacco, mold and other air bourn pollution exposure like carbon fuel exhaust from vehicles and airplanes. Lungs like Cannabis, it seems. Goodbye Asthma?

New Development: In Canada and England people who are sensitive to construction pollutants have a wonderful choice. Hemp Crete! Non psycho active Hemp aka Pot grows quickly and easily, an average house takes about three months of, is it three acres of growing? Hemp Crete is the product, building blocks twelve inches thick. No pollutants, slow burner, two hours to burn down, perfect insulation. Americans must pay extraordinarily to import Hemp Crete because we don't permit non psycho active Hemp growing in America. One such house is in Florida.

March 26,2013

Indians, Jews, Asians, Hispanics, Latinos and Latinas, Blacks, LGBTs, Fem-ales, Potheads. How does Society come to understand who is included? Rich and white? Rich? Well paid? Major athletes? Extreme talent or brains? Seen on TV? All the support people for same? All aspiring for inclusion who make the cut?

Imagine the plight of a Black Jewish Latina Lesbian Pothead in the middle 1980s. In Miami, not so bad.

The litmus test for included? Waspness. Money, Linage. Remember 'The Mayflower', as in came over on the first boat, Money. Royalty. Blue eyes? Blonde Hair? Not Catholic or Jewish but Protestant? It wasn't a Man's world as much as a White Man's world. The rest of us left conceding the duplicity of the upfront puritanical overtones, ostensibly moral, and the suspected hidden cheater's behaviors used to win the game of life materially.

Latest stock market brouhaha: Early April, 2014, The insidious mega taking of a tiny monetary advantage going to the fastest to buy to merely sell to the second, and so on. The first fast guy buys at the price immediately middle monning for profit a turnover sale to whomever is the second fast guy over and over for a big bucks return. The winner is the computer whose owner pays for it to chum up literally physically the closest to the computer with the price info, no humons involved. Can't be fair.

Picture an all 'white' populated red brick middle school in the late 1950's. See the open room cafeteria style lunchroom with long foldable tables. On each table sit tiny hollow elongated pyramids maybe three inches tall made of green construction grade paper folded to reveal three paragraphs of black print, each paragraph a prayer. One prayer appropriate for each, Catholic, Jewish, and Protestant. The folded cards sit in the center of every long table in the cafeteria in Woodrow Wilson Junior High, Tampa, Florida. The idea is to supply every child a prayer to say before that first bite. It proved inclusiveness, a hard won issue of the day.

Because one's church's pews may fill only with Wasps or whatever, one learns at school that religious equality rules. Islam is not big in America at this time.

In high school in the early 1960's we all took a required six week Americanism vs. Communism Class held in the auditorium. In retrospect, it appears the fear of the depth of penetration by the communists into our Society caused the need to propagandize teenagers.

The esteemed class for education about the American Way, inclusiveness, has to be Civics class. We learned in the ninth grade all about the United States Constitution, how it originated and what it gives us as American citizens along with our responsibilities and obligations to protect it's values on a person by person, citizen by citizen basis, with our voice and our vote. Choose Liberty and Justice.

<>*<><><>*<><><>*<><><>*<><><>*<>

The tune our culture has sung follows along lines of greed, hate, and hypocrisy. The tune for today and on is compassion, love, and generosity. War is NOT the answer. Peace is doable.

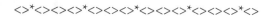

We learn that there are people for whom Ketamine, the horse tranquilizer, is an asset. They are a small number of us with certain disturbing behavioral characteristics. Ketamine makes a night and day improvement. To each their own.

We are evolving into a culture awakened into tolerance of other's choices for their own selves. Gays may marry. Be the person you are, newly free to openly love the person you love.

It may even mean equal legal status for same sex marriages soon. The future belongs to those who see freedom as our birthright start to finish.

Ideally the government will excuse itself from being involved in marriage licensing altogether. In the eyes of the government we shall be individuals birth to death. You may earn, be legally given, or inherit, parlay or sell assets to gain proceeds. You simply can't marry financial assets or liabilities. Wedding ceremonies will take off with conviction and commitment.

People may group. One by one, two by two, three by three, and so on. We may enjoin our friends and relatives to witness our union so they last for all time. Divorce ceremonies may facilitate closures. Choose your own take on a proper ceremony between you and your betrothed. Bring in the crowds or stand naked at home to make your union personally official. Hang a document of permanence on the wall. Match your rings and attire. Never part. Visit each other sporadically. Do legal name changing, every union is unique.

Wedding pageantry will flourish.

Religious marriage endorsement, great! Simply no government participation. Lawyers will write up the agreements. Or notarize and proceed. Beneficiaries shall be named for the usual. Nothing is automatic. Spousal and progeny inheritances must be legally defined. Simpler taxes, no hiding assets with a family member.

In the eyes of government, Federal, State and Local, we each remain an individual birth to death.

All agreements will be creatively individual. Child support remains legally enforced. Alimony would entail a document done ahead of the marriage fallout unless the breakup is done without animosity. Alimony or no alimony is agreed to as part of the break up, perhaps codified before a break.

No lawyers involved necessarily. You may acquire financial or other assets many ways, one simply may not marry to have them without a document saying so specifically. No two unions alike.

Children know no difference. Do your best by them and they will thrive. Once we are a Society operating without the confines of artifice to confound our natural changes and growth, talent and ambition for the goodness of life, we will blossom, emerging freely into the open. We may all thrive.

Marriage will come to embody loving and caring relationships only. No need to live a lie. Parents will become parents because a child is welcomed, when truth and justice rule. Marriage isn't an institution. It is a particular satisfying union forged by those partaking and prolonged by that self same satisfaction. Let's celebrate and enjoy familial happiness as it is surely meant to be enjoyed, honestly and openly. No shackles.

Wandered off subject. Tangential thinking is one of the noticed possible results of a good high. Given time and place a bit of THC becomes a mind opening experience.

Warning: Momentary loss of any warm fuzziness.

One wonders if that nineteen year old Boston Marathon bomber hadn't ceased his chill factor weeks ahead of Monday, Patriot's Day, April 15, 2013. He did alter his trajectory weeks ahead of his most horrific act we are told over National Public Radio. A Chill is a colloquialism like Stoner or Pothead. Pothcads are said to be mellow, less excitable.

Chilled out does not connote anything resembling a person likely to act out as dangerous in a deadly suicidal hurt your own, killer of innocent people, kind of way. Good cover.

Supposition: These killers lived a double life. One on the surface, another as cunning as any underground with a façade, maybe. Then a break out, they, the brothers et.al. pour their passionate hatred out.

Thankfully we hear of the boundless goodness that makes ever growing ripples of wonders and goodness the harvest reaped from The Boston Marathon 2013.

u24u24u24u24u24u24u24u24u24u24u

Hypocrisy by definition: The United States Government, The Feds, supply medical Marihuana to four Americans. Yes, our United States Government supplies four Americans their Pot. This heard on NPR, National Public Radio, WKED, New York, Monday April 22,2013, Earth Day, mid afternoon show. The Speaker related first hand knowledge of four individuals who are supplied Pot by our Federal Government as the remnants of those who have received medicinal Pot from the government under a by name, Compassionate Plan, begun in 1992 to relieve these specific people's suffering.

The male speaker told about a person who is a well respected financial advisor who always smokes a joint right before doing her show and is brilliant. Another Federal Pot smoker is a very successful New York Stock Exchange Hedge

Fund Manager who smokes a joint outside with the tobacco users on breaks. Another man goes about a full normal life smoking Pot consistently and continuously. He carries a card that may be read by an Official with a need to know he's legal. His bones are diseased. The speaker also said one of his subjects in this reveal of the government's own Potheads takes breaks from Pot for a period of time occasionally.

Unfortunately the I-Pad App lost signal for more of this NPR Radio Broadcast reminder and update of a long ago United States Government ability to allow a Creation Given Natural Resource Health Restorative and Superior Libation besides being an Environmentally Advantageous Herb, to be legal to those with proof galore of the night and day difference with THC relief, nothing else comparing.

Naturally this begs the question of why is Pot a Schedule I Classification Felonious Drug. A Schedule I Classification requires a drug so classified to show no medicinal purpose and be dangerous to use. Say what?

Where is the paper trail showing the documentation of creation of this scheme of Classification? Who did this Classification in the first place?

Pot isn't dangerous yet is rich in medicinal purpose.

Cigarettes start fires and kill users. Enough said.

ZZZ#Z#Z#Z#ZZ#ZZ#ZZ#ZZZ

As recently as early in the year 2013, there was a court ruling re-endorsing the erroneous classification of Pot. It was the Federal Appeals Court in Washington, D.C. and done summarily. Details in the next pages.

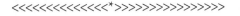

The obvious option to reclassify Pot as not felonious is one of the choices in a list of options mentioned on these pages for a legal sidestep to end the unproductive for the Common Good, No Just Cause, Persecution of Potheads.

Options for legalizing non persecution:

A. <u>Employ the Severality Clause</u>, [See 185 this book] The Severality Clause poses two Avenues:

1). <u>Unenforceable</u>: Truth, the never convicted as felon folk may sit at home not buying, not selling, not growing, smoking pot? Yes. Simply keep your garbage free of evidence, apply strategies for most humon non detection, conceal your stash consistently. Watch for tell tale breath. Eat. Wash.

Here's an unconfirmed diagnosis of our literally existent drug crime hierarchy; in one's owned, mortgaged or rented castle or hovel one may freely smoke. There's no law against it. If, however, you are in public and have contraband itself in plain sight, or if you are victimized by a narcotics alert dog, a sniffer dog or otherwise detected, or if the police walk in with or without a warrant into your castle and your stash or paraphernalia is found or in plain sight, trouble.

Stash and accoutrements hidden, smoke in the air, no warrant, you're okay. Don't be persuaded to let the police in your door without a warrant signed by a judge, gently. Look at the warrant and get names and badge numbers if you can. Post No Trespassing signs before this happens. End of unconfirmed diagnosis.

2). <u>Exceptions are acceptable</u> if you, Congress, say so.

<u>B</u>. Supreme Court announces decision to frame out their plan to recognize the nation has a willingness to allow legal Pot for medicinal purposes in addition to placing a hold on punitive actions against recreational use.

<u>C</u>. Without so much as a by your leave the laws against Pot evaporate off the books, effectively speaking. Unspoken Non Enforcement Policy, Like the laws against cohabitation, formally dropped as recently as early 2013 in West Virginia.

<u>D</u>. President makes proclamation of freedom for the non criminals in our prisons. Ipso facto we have defacto legalization.

Truth is, this cat left the bag a looooong time ago.

Time to straighten our posture in the world. Show true leadership and genuine compassion for the people who do and will avail themselves of the stupidly forbidden asset to the Humon Condition, dear Pot.

Cease the Hypocrisy United States Government. Choose Compassion. It's not enough you have a law that supports bigotry and prejudice. You have to prove you have a just cause to the rest of us.

To all those who are constituent vote job dependent, two words to the wise: Tread gently. You'll find that Potheads are people that are loved and respected by friends, co-workers and relatives, same as everybody. Potheads are said to be eight percent of everybody in America, roughly twenty eight million people and counting.

Recap: 2014 marks One hundred years of persecution. The Harrison Act of 1914 did nothing but harm to the opiate addicts who were summarily made criminals. Doctors and pharmacists had worked to help addicts ready to stop the habit and treated others. The Harrison Act of 1914 also made criminals of those persisting treating addicts. In three months the number of people addicted to narcotics tripled. Help forbidden.

The underworld codified, tax free profits beckoned, enhancing the shower of untold power and wealth on outlaws.

The legal, eighteenth amendment placed on our constitution, the Alcohol Prohibition of thirteen years, 1919 to 1933, created tax free mammoth dollars. Mega wealth pocketed moving the illegal liquid libation in such demand. From the 1930's Pot is demonized to the public in movies produced by a pharmaceutical empire bent on the public buying their lab pills, at the onset, Bayer aspirin. Next came the Narcotics Tax Act of 1937 and opps! Pot is swept in and outlawed. Result, minorities are the clear target for law enforcement to jail. Prejudice enjoys the showy centerpiece of a white supremacy culture in the 1930s. It's Wealth and Power popularized and imposed world wide.

The Drug Abuse Prevention and Control - 1970 Law took over and has been added to steadily to 2010. Read the chronological rundown of the over thirty Acts of Congress added to same, Pages 116 and 117, this book.

At no point in the entire last one hundred years has drug illegality served the public. Drug Wars, pointless. Ours is very well tax payer funded escapades designed to run the prices up on street drugs at best(?) and at worst, scare half the population into fear of being caught in the crossfire. The as yet unidentified villain of the piece? Our cupidity at being so manipulated by the moneyed. No more. Persecution is persecution no matter how familiar and tolerated. Slavery went down. Jews beloved. Drug War persecution perpetuates, promulgates and enhances crime. We are our own victims, whether conned into a user, living on the wrong side of the law, or doing the persecution, we all pay for our unenlightened behaviors and viewpoints.

Imagine now the world without the lie of persecution as justice. . . .

Los Angeles, has decided to eliminate one hundred thirty five of it's eight hundred pot dispensaries. They were more ubiquitous than Starbucks, so something had to be done. Story reported by National Public Radio May 23rd 2012. The American Broadcast Company, ABC television, is airing a similar story of an over run by Pot town early November 4th, 2013. The promotional advertising on local southwest Florida ABC TV is to suit the local advertisers and is also set in California. This to win over the hearts and minds of those willing to allow this to happen to Florida. This being more Pot dispensaries than Starbucks in a given place. And what, exactly, is wrong about that?

Why not work out intelligent Regulations as this change unfolds?

A television commercial offers business owners the opportunity to have a sniffer dog. Dogs are easily trained to detect any smell, we hear. Hazardous Narcotics, oils, a list is cited for example, May 23rd, 2013. So many dog handlers and the government are obliging to 'bear down' on Potheads and the rest. The Supreme Court so far not ruling against or in favor of residential front door dog sniffing. The police are asking to allow a trained sniffer dog to legally be brought to any front door to signal by sitting to alert their handler/enforcement officer of the presence of an offending odor or stay standing and try next door where again the dog will sniff the doorknob.

Drug Court History:

Drug Court began in Dade County Florida in the nineteen eighties. Illegal Drug providers were in and out and back in again, and repeat back again, into the local busy judicial system. The potential innocence of the Marihuana drug trade and consumers didn't occur at the time. Along with the then Florida Attorney General, Janet Reno, Dade County legislators formulated a treatment enforcement plan with Drug Court personnel supervision. Interventions, group therapy, counseling ensued along with mandatory court appearances for the "clients". Pee tests. Mess up? More Drug Court ordered treatment or days in jail.

The stated intention of Drug Court is to reduce regular crime. 'Drugs' are assumed to be a close tie to criminal behavior. That is the idea behind making drugs contraband, obviously? Since growing, buying and selling and publicly using pot are all no-nos, Drug Court clientele is often as innocent of actual crime as the court personnel. It's erroneously assumed there's a teachable improvement to be made by counseling Potheads. In the 1970s New York City programs for Pot offenders had to be abandoned due to the quality life performance level of Potheads. Potheads are good people, too.

A Pothead without the stigma of lawlessness is as fully productive and functional as anyone.

Aside: It would be nice to use some of the latest paraphernalia thus avoiding the short pipe with it's close to the inhalation point hot lighter flame.

The government is directly responsible for prohibiting an asset for the humon condition from being sold in it's best presentations from edibles to inhalers.

Also mentioned as a general intention of Drug Court is checking for substance abuse related disease. Seems like a perhaps helpful outcome. Health care with out a turn with handcuffs would work even more efficiently.

Fuss over a no abuse ridden, proven medicinal Herb? When drug abuse has swung to laboratory/manufactured pain killers away from opiates and back. The tracking of prescription drugs seems an easy supply to trace back. That seems like the solution recently employed. The underworld answering back with cocaine then heroin to the unsuspecting looking to fill the scripted drug void. No visibility. No accountability. Disposable middlemun are waiting in line.

A small town Drug Court was written up in the paper with a story proclaiming how beneficial Drug Court is to whole families. Maybe so. Is help handcuffs and loss of Liberty? Reformulate to be truly respectful help without the literal or metaphoric face in the dirt to start.

The Drug Court Concept began in the 1980's Miami area and had success processing the huge population of baby boomer individuals that could be rounded up visibly using, buying or selling, or conveying or growing contra banded drugs.

Miami's Drug Court success got around the country.

The above reference is part of the 12th Circuit Court, State of Florida, and United States Programs Services, as per the Drug Court Appendix's online article titled <u>Breaking the Cycle Between Drugs and Crime.</u>

Currently, May 28, 2013, two thousand and six hundred Drug Courts, numbers swelling, are busy. The point of Drug Court is to shunt clients into drug free lives. Why not shunt the alcoholics before they maim and kill? Or shunt the nicotine addicts into stringent programs so the one third of them don't die of tobacco use and so much illness in innocent bystanders disappears. Two extremely harmful physiologically addictive poisonous 'Drugs'! The user is harmed and the non using innocent are harmed. It does not get worse than that. Questions? Keep reading.

Where is the respect for Medicinal and Recreational Pot use? The residents of twenty states are finding out. No more jail time for Potheads. Twenty states and Washington DC. have spoken.

The twenty legal Pot states are arguably feasible enough precedent for Nationwide application. Let Freedom Ring! One Union, Under God!

<> PROHIBITION <>

The Alcohol Prohibition began as ratified January 16,1919. It ended thirteen years later as repealed December 5,1933. Two thirds of our state legislatures voted to add the eighteenth amendment and then, by convention voted to repeal the Alcohol Prohibition amendment from our original and fundamental document, the United States Constitution. Of all twenty seven amendments to our Constitution, one prohibits proximity to alcohol, intoxicating liquor, as illegal. That's the eighteenth amendment. The twenty first amendment legalized and regulated intoxicating liquors as a controlled substance.

Alcohol was a legal across the board Prohibition. The Congressional Acts passed by Congress, lack the legal authority to suspend individual rights without a JUST CAUSE.

Across the board, every person seeking relief or uplift from a God Given Natural Resource Health Restorative and Superior Libation is criminalized at the point of acquisition. Some less than others starting January 1, 2014, since recreational use of Pot passed as law in Washington State and Colorado last November, 2012.

Our United States Congress may not subject to arbitrary criminality a swath of us, not by skin color, not by heritage, not by Herbal preferences, not one of, or all of, so many innocent people. Congress may not make criminal a subset of the population. Prosecutors have yet to prove their case against the innocent choosing Marijuana en mass.

Congress cannot convey the right to trespass to remove an innocent individual from their liberty in the case of Cannabis. Do we seek to lock up intoxicating liquor imbibers where they drink? There a case is easily made. The killing and maiming of the unsuspecting by drunk drivers, domestic violence, mental and physical deterioration. And likewise nicotine addicts, creating so much expense, pain and sorrow.

These are two detrimental potentially fatal substances, legal substances.

All these groups have a guarantee made by the United States Constitution. Yet our Congress is unconstitutionally complicit year after year continuing persecution by prosecution and the threat of prosecution. No viable criminality exists to point to. Neither ingesting individuals or the vegetation Marijuana before consumption are a nuisance. Both individuals and the vegetation deserve law enforcement service and protection.

Law enforcement prosecution makes no case beyond the unjust so called law which in reality is an erroneous policy. Trespass arrests take almost a million American individuals a year into the system, the arresting officers in violation of the to be arrestee's personal space. The law/policy, blatantly violates eight percent plus, about twenty eight million Americans' right to Choose Pot. The result? Many individuals' right to life, liberty and the pursuit of happiness, aborted.

There is never an acceptable excuse to discriminate against innocent people. Potheads want on the proverbial Bus.

ahuhahuhahuhahuhahuhahuha

Late August 2013 serves up another Presidential Nugget. President Obama announces the Federal Policy for Prosecutors in the states who have legalized Pot for medicinal use and the two recreational Pot use states, making twenty states plus Washington, the District of Columbia. The consumer of medicinal and small amounts of recreation Pot may now do so free of the fear of a raid or arrest. Huge! It's an eight point memo of reasonable conditions.

Some of those Prosecutors are quickly pushing back with some saying, "No." In practice no such problems have arisen by April 5,2014.

@@@@@@@@@@@@@@@@@@@@@@@@

Isn't it the job of the Drug Enforcement Agency to provide the negative or criminal aspects of a Schedule I Classified Drug? It is the most felonious category for a controlled substance. No, they are waiting on proven medicinal efficacy. The appeals court said that's right, 2013. It's a Catch 22. Monkey business. Cannabis is proven medicinally efficient, just not to them, for shame.

Cannabis has a clean history as an asset for the humon condition.

The DEA says they lack knowledge of any efficacy study of Cannabis to substantiate Cannabis as having medical benefits. Therefore it remains a felony to be caught possessing Cannabis even in a meager amount in thirty states. Or to grow, or move about. Having consumed, no problem unless you drive badly. Then you could experience double trouble.

When will truth and justice count the most?

))))))))))))))))))))))))))))

FALSE:
1. Not according with truth or fact; incorrect; not according with rules of law.
2. appearing to be the thing denoted; deliberately made or meant to deceive. artificial; feigned. 3. illusionary; not actually so.

PREMISE:
Logic a previous or proposition from which another is inferred or follows as a conclusion; an assertion or proposition that forms the basis for a work or theory (premise something on/upon) base an argument, theory or under taking on: *the reforms were premised on our findings.* state or presuppose (something) as a premise: [with cause] *one thought premised that the cosmos is indestructible.*

{AS PER *The Oxford American College Dictionary based on The New Oxford American Dictionary. Published in 2001, as published thusly in 2002}*

SCHEDULE I Drugs, (United States) from Wikipedia
To be a Schedule I drug under the Controlled Substances Act for the United States:
Required findings for drugs to be placed in this Schedule:

1. The drug or other substance has a high potential for abuse
2. The drug or other substance has no currently accepted medical use in treatment in the United States.
3. There is a lack of accepted safety for use of the drug or other substance under medical supervision.

Except as specifically authorized, it is illegal for any person:

1. To manufacture, distribute, or dispense, or possess with the intent to manufacture, distribute, or dispense, a controlled substance; or
2. To create, distribute, or dispense, or possess with intent to distribute or dispense, a counterfeit substance.

Review Online: List of Schedule I drugs (US) under hallucinogenic or psychedelic substances, as

Tetrahydrocannabinol (THC) numbered 7370

Hereby and Henceforth the people demand the government defend it's intrusion into anyone's life to relieve them of their liberty over Cannabis. Prove Cannabis bad. Provide a JUST CAUSE substantiating the non imbibers superiority or the imbibers inferiority. Not for one or two or this one and that one, but a general all Cannabis arrest Unifying Just Cause. Primary Court criminality, existing in current law, a law whose purpose is to protect all Americans from criminal behavior perpetrators. That is the standard for an offence being an offence. In fact each Cannabis arrest is an offence to all citizens. This is America. The government doesn't run the people. The people run the government.

###

"Without any resisting you, officer," [Be a citizen in good standing to make a citizen's arrest of the officer(s)]

"I make a citizen's arrest of you based on your intrusion into my life to relieve me of my liberty. You have no Just Cause. Your action is based on a false premise. Unacceptable. A Just Cause must be proven, yet cannot be. I am one of twenty eight million Americans plus who know Cannabis is an asset to the humon condition. Therefore I make a citizen's arrest of you Officer(s)for intruding into my life to relieve me of my liberty without Just Cause."

Go over the officer's Miranda rights:

"You have the right to remain silent. What you say and do can and will be used against you in a court of law. You have the right to legal representation. If you can not afford legal representation the court will appoint legal representation for you."

###

Truth: Sniffer dogs and pee tests for Cannabis (THC) detection are both invasions, falsely premised. Both sniffer dogs and pee tests actually prove the case for the innocence of Cannabis in the lives of American people. No observable criminality with our humon perceptions. No, a dog's ultra sensitive nose or a lab manufactured test of one's own urine is the accuser. No crime, no off behavior, no implicit risking of the innocent, nothing.

Pee Tests are an invasion of privacy and amount to forcing a person to abandon their Fifth Amendment right not to incriminate themselves.

This is America where the people are not subjected to tyranny.

Let's make it so. Potheads are people too, good people.

+!+!+!+!+!+!+!+!+!+!+!+!+!+!+

October 3, 2013 is the third day of a huge Federal Government shutdown of the non essential. It's drastic.

The Tea Party Republicans have gone off the deep end. All of everything funded by Federal annual funds, except our troops, an exception as is Medicare and such, shut down. Many children are not fed at school, daycares are closed, National Parks, Bureaucratic offices of all manner locked. It's dire and expensive. The reason for the contrary behavior is Republican opposition in Congress to the Affordable Health Care Act, a legal and popular law passed to provide affordable health care to Americans. Yes, a penalty is owed with opting out. The Tea Partiers hate Obamacare, their name for the AHC Act.

The United States House of Representatives is a majority Republican Congress currently, by a squeak. The leadership of the majority, Senator Boehner, is with the Tea Partiers on the shutting down. They want a year delay on the now three day old initial phase start up of the Affordable Health Care Act because they know the people will, we the people will, fight to keep it if once having it. The thirty Tea Partiers, refuse to take a long delay and other mean spirited tactics off the table.

Disgust at Republicans is universal unless you are sitting pretty financially AND lack compassion.

Of course the President had a Continuing Resolution to sign into law in his hands just after midnight the midnight of October 17th an allowable few minutes late. The morning of the 18th dawned with furloughed federal employees off to work, business as usual. Undesirable repercussions are accessed from the sixteen day, mostly all of the federal government Shut Down.

Most Americans are attributing the shut down and it's bad outcomes to the bullying done by the Representative

Ted Cruz adherents. The House of Representatives made a new rule of order to disallow anyone but Representative Eric Cantor to ask for a vote on the floor of the house. Majority Leader Boehner swayed himself into the no-vote-called camp because that would end the Shut Down against Ted's wishes.

The way the Shut Down ended? Finally, a vote on the floor. It took place days and days past having had the same result only mercifully before the onset of the shut down, for goodness sakes.

Voters in the polling booth could fix this mess. Look to the 2014 mid term elections.

To do: Vote 2014 to legalize medical Marihuana, Floridians. Sign up to make it so. Florida Attorney General Pam Bondi announces seeking to stop the medical Marihuana referendum from being on the ballot November, 2014. November 1, 2014 Bondi says the wording on the proposed referendum is misleading to the public. The Florida State Supreme Court is to rule. At that same date, the first of November, two hundred thousand signatures on the petition for legalizing Pot are in place. A minimum of seven hundred thousand are required some time in February 2014, or by February. December 2013, five hundred signatures are on the Petition.

The arguments have been heard. We wait.

We are advised to contact our state legislators with our input. Ask for Freedom to replace persecution. Say we the people demand the state legislature pass a law legalizing medical Marihuana immediately and set a date in 2014 to legalize recreational Pot as well.

Such a legalizing bill is tendered in Florida's legislature. It went to committee and isn't likely to get out. March, 2014.

The Huffington Post researched and provided the public with this list of 18 Milestones That Led To Our Marijuana "Tipping Point"

Here are the 18 steps in synopsis, chronologically reordered:

1. The Marihuana plant is used medicinally in China 10,000 years ago. It's uses multifold; rope, paper, clothing, medicine.

2. Our American founding fathers are big on Hemp, making sails, lamp oil.

3. Late 19th century Pot is sold from stores in Mexico. [Key West and more, too] In 1910 the Mexican Revolution sent immigrants with Marijuana over the border making some Americans aware of Pot as an asset. Others saw Pot as tainted by the immigrant Mexicans linked with crime, stigmatizing Marijuana.

4. Cannabis in production in America diminishes to nothing by the 1960s over an anti -'drug' mainstream mindset. [Negative Aggression defeated Marijuana as market place competition starting with the Narcotics Act of 1937, erroneously including Marijuana.] Synthetic fibers won. [Phamaceuticals and alcohol sales won too.] By 1967, the Beetles, The Fab Four, were revolutionizing the world. Marijuana is embraced by young adults everywhere in America and abroad.

5. 1973 Oregon reduces the penalty for Marijuana possession. The Shafer Commission endorses legalizing small Marijuana amounts. Then President, Richard Nixon, rejects the endorsment. NORML, the National Organization for the Reform of Marijuana Law. is begun. Cheech and Chong as hugely popular comedians in the movies, take Marijuana familiarity a significant leap forward.

6. Starting in 1974, High Times, the magazine, grows knowledge of and support for Marijuana and it is still publishing.

7. Glaucoma afflicted Robert Randall is a Federally legally prescribed Marihuana user growing his own in Washington D.C. since 1975. He won.

8. The first city to legally give medical patients access to Marijuana? San Francisco in 1991.

9. California, 1996, legalizes cultivating and possessing Marijuana for medical treatment.

10. Now there are twenty states and the District of Columbia that have passed medical Marijuana law.

11. Cancer metastasis stops with treatment with a Marijuana compound, as discovered by two scientists in San Francisco. Other scientists in the United Kingdom find Marijuana compounds treat leukemia.

12. Cannabis [Marijuana] Oil is credited with successfully eliminating seizures from three hundred a week to three in eight months for a six year old, Charlotte Figi.

13. Colorado and Washington State pass recreational use of Marijuana, November Elections 2012. Recreational Marijuana shops to open 2014.

14. August, 2013, Attorney General Eric Holder tells Washington and Colorado to create the bureaucracy to run regulation and implementation for the legal use of Marijuana for adults.

15. Kentucky legalizes industrial Hemp production early in 2013. North Dakota and West Virginia also have Hemp laws.

16. 2013, a farmer in Colorado grows and harvests a Hemp crop, the first since 1957 in this country.

17. Marijuana, the Cannabis business, is said to be arriving big time.

    Investors see huge opportunity and are acting. Projections show sales of legal Marijuana will exceed global smart phone sales.

18. Polling shows more Americans than ever, now more than fifty-eight percent, agree Marijuana should be legal. Up from fifty percent in 2011.

    Thanks Huffington Post! Yes. Marihuana is good for the economy as well as individuals.

A new court is evolving. A Buffalo New York Judge, Robert Russell, created a Veterans Treatment Court, per say, in 2008. He gave them their own docket adding many experts and agencies for improved outcomes. The judge focused attention on each individual with donated and tax payer funded time and service. His court demonstrates an outstanding application of compassion. His system is catching on due to the recognition of the special trama the Veteran offenders generally have suffered and continue to suffer. As heard on NPR, National Public Radio November, 2013. There are fifty eight courts like it.

Perhaps we will evolve that level of compassion to include everyone's someone.

Nelson Mandela, who served twenty seven consecutive years incarcerated for actively pushing for the end of apartheid, recently died and is laid to rest December 14, 2013 in the small home village of his youth. Of course his life is revered for his being and his part ending apartheid. There's no more official segregation of whites from everybody else in the country of South Africa. His part in spreading the truth of equality of individuals no matter their skin color will remain significant into eternity.

At this time apartheid exists all over the world. Women are held apart from education and opportunity. Education legitimately qualifies, or it's lack eliminates, individuals from employment. The notion that our United States Congress has the right to set Marihuana aficionados, or any substance adherents aside as criminal individuals legally, is wrong. The by passing of the required two thirds of all our states' state legislatures to ratify an amendment to the United Sates Constitution, is in and of itself unconstitutional. We live under apartheid by indefensible policy.

Indefensible morally, indefensible legally, indefensible by outcome is the apartheid that incarcerates Marihuana growers, traffickers, buyers and sellers. Users are victims if caught in public where the police are.

You, the readers, now have the knowledge to speak out and vote for truth and justice. Law is evolutionary. It just wants enough people who abhor the dishonesty of persecution of innocent Marihuana aficionados. That dishonesty directly enhances the sale of the toxic, potentially quite lethal drugs, alcohol, tobacco, and pharmaceutical lab drugs. This while creating inane warring with deaths by gunfire. It creates drug lord territories. It fills our jails with the persecuted. Ultimately we are each denied the known and unknown advantages of a proven asset to the humon condition, Marijuana.

Marihuana is an environmentally friendly, creation given, health restorative and superior libation. Marihuana also has much to offer as an industrial fiber, for example Hemp Crete building blocks for non-allergenic homes with a three hour burn down time and more.

Let's teach our Congress to respect the individual as having inalienable rights to pursue happiness. Let there be no more lumping us as disposable huddled masses of fodder ripe for big business manipulation and exploitation. The law is on the side of truth of justice. We have only to make it so.

Dishonest vs. Honest. The blanket supposition all Pot consumers are dishonest criminal types is laughable. Laugh yourself to tears. The injustice served up wholesale for all Americans and the rest of the people of the world all but smothers the life out of truth and therefore mutual trust.

Who in this everlasting, so far, hundred year war whose net result is all consuming growth of crime and suffering benefiting? Not We the People. We are not served or protected by paying for our own oppression and persecution.

The misguided notion that the 'drug' consumer is responsible for the bloodshed of the Drug War is a notion for the misguided and ignorant. Include consumers of every ilk possible for no one persuasion works for all. No one people may speak for all. It's Liberty and Justice for all, right?

Legal Smoke-In in Seattle, Oregon! Money motivates investment. Society is pushed to regroup. Story unfolding. BBC World News America, December 16, 2013. Marihuana acceptance is quickly taking over here in the country that gave us the Drug War.

Discriminating against a person's Skin Color and Discriminating against the people liking Pot, are both the SAME, in that both are based on a False Notion of Superiority. People liking Pot are not just persecuted but are the victims of a Federal Hate Crime, a State level Hate Crime, and Local Law Enforcement Hate Crime, to put a Fine Point on it.

No evidence exists to excuse or make sense of contra banding Cannabis much less to relieve citizens of their liberty over it. To say the Drug Enforcement Agency, aka the DEA, not having an acceptable Study in the courtroom (January,

2013) to substantiate the Efficacy of Medical Marihuana is reason enough to maintain the Status Quo of all manner of Incarceration and Ruin spread Globally, encompassing the Innocent and shaping Negative Cultures, IS NUTS!

Don't Advocate for Anyone to use Pot.
Advocate for Everyone to have the Choice.

Floridians will decide yea or nay to Medical Marijuana November, 2014.

February 28, 2014. Marijuana this and Marihuana that. Every media business has covered extensively the coming to a head of this explosive new industry. Colorado? Say Pot Rush. Visit as a rich tourist and be Limoed and dined housed and feted all with the best Pot at your disposal. Pay cash.

Banks are snubbing the Pot trade making this a monumental issue for seller/growers. If you sell Pot in Colorado legitimately you grow it too. If you buy Pot legitimately in Colorado you may also pay tax as high as thirty six percent.

"There's gold in them there buds!" Colorado is getting rich.

Congress? Still so polarized the irrelevance of the one side stymies the other side. Tea Party Representative Ryan talks impeachment of President Obama. No traction possible.

Ryan's mouth gave us one more moment of idiotic distraction, a Tea Party basic and always lame tactic.

The Congressional Democrats attempt to create jobs funding education and infrastructure to make our country back into a top notch country. Our children are less proficient than others over the world scholastically. We've fallen behind on reducing infant mortality. There are so many aspects missing of what it takes to churn out the innovators and world class leadership to keep us with our competitive edge on the global stage. We allow hunger and homelessness to persist. We are on track to visit Mars with devices.

Wait! Saturn has a moon with what appears(?) to be an Ocean of H2O hidden under a large portion of the Saturn moon surface. News of a life sustaining element for possible exploration, April 3,2014. You just never know.

The health care mega industry is gearing up to derail Marijuana and is doomed to failure. Truth and Justice get trampled routinely but their staying power trumps even the glossiest of campaigns. The side down with reality seeks Truth and Justice and can not fail to win. Mega manipulation of our choices? Over.

A spokesperson for the Drug Enforcement Agency or another government auspices heard televised March 24, 2014 on C-span mentioned our government, our Federal Government, was not pursuing for arrest the adult final consumers of Marihuana. The concern is to keep our adolescents off Pot because it is dangerous to our young people's brains. The spokesperson said it causes drops in Intelligent Quotient points in developing adolescent brains. He sited no study and referenced no source for this statement.

Imagine the parents of the many adolescents whose life ended in a car crash, the young driver drunk on alcohol. Beyond dangerous, deadly. Picture the under eighteen year old hooked on nicotine looking at a sickly shortened life set to cost us all financially and hampering the well being of family, friends and strangers with second and third hand smoke. Obviously Marihuana substituted for the deadly drugs in both these scenarios would render a blissful outcome comparatively.

Changing alcoholic drunkenness from it's status as rite of passage to adulthood and dumping totally on the sexiness of cigarette smoking? Now there would be two quantum leaps forward for our mutual cultural health and happiness. Keeping Marihuana illegal? Just plain dumb.

You go get 'em Pot Heads of the world. The truth is out. Marijuana is a tremendous asset to the humon condition. Meanwhile Colorado's law enforcement is to be taught the tells of a stoned individual because a Pot high is not detectable like drunkenness.

Profiling strikes again. Use that Visine so your eyes aren't red. If confronted be serious, no exuberance. Prepare ahead of driving, have no detectable Pot breath or Pot resin on your hands. One is not in private in a vehicle.

So what are the tells? Better reaction time, better focus, more stamina, slower driving?

Ladies and Gentlemun we embark on a new era. It is not good versus evil, not right versus wrong. Truth and justice reveal Marijuana as a beneficial Herb for all humonkind and a natural resource for industry. Marijuana supports no controversy in the final analysis. The nay sayers will lose eight Intelligence Quotient points persisting in unsubstantiated claims of Intelligence Quotient dropping eight points for young Pot Heads. Not nine, not seven?

Makes you wonder. Beware the talking heads that talk in absolutes. It's propaganda, and not the good kind.

Lastly, consider this: Knowing what we know commonly now about Marijuana; no deaths, medically effective, outcomes so superior to tobacco and alcohol use. We must each be outraged our tax dollars pay to incarcerate growers, traffickers and vendors. Users handcuffed, arrested and forced into court without a defense. Evidently consumer arrests will now be done by ignorant state and local law enforcement only, it appears. Don't smoke Pot publicly.

The Modern Draconian Era begun one hundred years ago in February 1914 must end. Peace and Understanding are meant to rule the world. Getting past keeping Cannabis illegal is the measure of our ability to succeed as a people. Truth and Justice or Arcane Stupidity and Greed, you choose.

Stupidity: n
1. lack of intelligence: lack of intelligence, perception, or common sense
2. rashness or thoughtlessness: extremely rash or thoughtless behavior

Encarta ® World English Dictionary © & (P) 1998-2005 Microsoft Corporation. All rights reserved.

Truth: n
1. -something factual: the thing that corresponds to fact or reality
   If you tell the truth, you have nothing to fear.
   -spoke the truth.
2. true quality: correspondence to fact or reality
3. true statement: a statement that corresponds to fact or reality
   His story was a mixture of truths and untruths.
4. obvious fact: something that is so clearly true that it hardly needs to be stated
5. something generally believed: a statement that is generally believed to be true, a religious truth
6. honesty: honesty and sincerity
   I can say in all truth that I never knew about his crimes.
7. conformity: adherence to a standard or law

8. loyalty: faithfulness to a person or a cause (dated)
9. U.K. accuracy: accuracy of alignment, setting, position, or shape (dated)

[Old English trēowth "faithfulness" < trēow (see true)]
Encarta ® World English Dictionary © & (P) 1998-2005 Microsoft Corporation. All rights reserved.

Justice: n
1. fairness: fairness or reasonableness, especially in the way people are treated or decisions are made
2. system or application of law: the legal system, or the act of applying or upholding the law
3. validity: validity in law
4. good reason: sound or good reason
5. judge: a judge, especially of a higher court

[12th century. Via French < Latin justitia < justus (see just)]

Bring somebody to justice to arrest somebody to be tried in a court of law

Do justice to somebody or something to deal with somebody or something fairly to convey the true qualities, especially the merits, of somebody or something

Do yourself justice to display your own abilities fully or perform to your full potential (often used in the negative)
Encarta ® World English Dictionary © & (P) 1998-2005 Microsoft Corporation. All rights reserved.

Epilogue

Amazingly the Tampa Bay Times, the newspaper of St. Petersburg, Florida, presented on their April 13, 2014 Sunday edition Front Page, top and bottom, a story entitled <u>Wired to work with Marijuana?</u> The article featured drawn graphics illustrating a humon brain and another showing a humon body shape indicating locations of the THC receptors through out the body and most specifically the brain. Substantiation of built in THC receptors. Indeed. Biologist and author Gregory Gerdeman's <u>The Pot Book: A Complete Guide to Cannabis</u> provided the factual input for the story. Unfortunately the comeuppance of this revealed knowledge provided in the newspaper article appeared to promote the concept of new isolatable chemicals to make new lab drugs for doctors to administer. The strongest resonance of the timely article, however, is that Marijuana is a natural resource proven as an intended, far reaching benefit to the humon body, mind and soul. Apparently THC is welcomed by the many receptors spread out over our bodies. It offers a way for the mechanics of anxiety, pain, inflammation, lots of negatives to not spin into cell burn out. It's a save yourself from frayed nerves etc. medicine. It hampers crucial cells from damaging. Common knowledge at last.

Thank you.

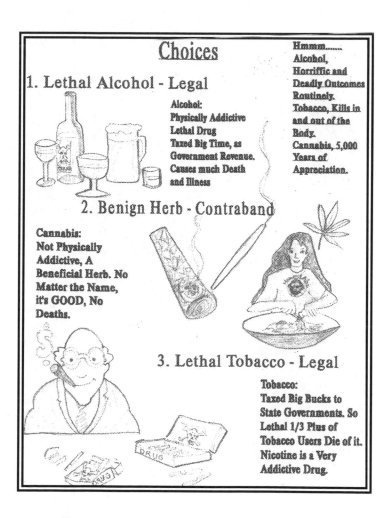

Choices

Hmmm.......
Alcohol,
Horriffic and
Deadly Outcomes
Routinely.
Tobacco, Kills in
and out of the
Body.
Cannabis, 5,000
Years of
Appreciation.

1. Lethal Alcohol - Legal

Alcohol:
Physically Addictive
Lethal Drug
Taxed Big Time, as
Government Revenue.
Causes much Death
and Illness

2. Benign Herb - Contraband

Cannabis:
Not Physically
Addictive, A
Beneficial Herb. No
Matter the Name,
it's GOOD, No
Deaths.

3. Lethal Tobacco - Legal

Tobacco:
Taxed Big Bucks to
State Governments. So
Lethal 1/3 Plus of
Tobacco Users Die of it.
Nicotine is a Very
Addictive Drug.

Author's Privilege Remark: Words to the wise.

A ttention all men! For the best outcomes reproductively speaking please cease consumption of all toxins and poisons six months before embarking on conception of your child and fatherhood. No alcohol, no pharmaceuticals, or even tobacco, nothing to compromise the development of your sperm when it forms in you. Please search online the words Sperm Division to understand how much exposure there is to your content as a sperm is made. Sperm live up to six months.

Wemun have a similar responsibility for the health of a fetus and future child with one difference. There is a five day window before the fertilized egg attaches to a womon's blood stream for nutrients. Over all health of a mother to be does impact the child and consumption of toxins is a no-no through out gestation and nursing. The same six months of consumption preparation for conception is also recommended for mothers.

Thank you.